Women, health and medicine

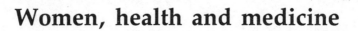

Agnes Miles

Open University Press
Milton Keynes · Philadelphia

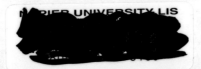

Open University Press
Celtic Court
22 Ballmoor
Buckingham
MK18 1XW

and
1900 Frost Road, Suite 101
Bristol, PA 19007, USA

First Published 1991
Reprinted 1992, 1993

British Library Cataloguing in Publication Data

Miles, Agnes
    Women, health and medicine.
    I. Title
    362.1082

    ISBN 0–335–09906–8
    ISBN 0–335–09905–X pbk

Library of Congress Cataloging-in-Publication Data

Miles, Agnes.
      Women, health, and medicine/Agnes Miles.
         p.   cm.
      Includes bibliographical references and index.
      ISBN 0–335–09906–8 (hardback) – ISBN 0–335–09905–X (pbk.)
      1. Women – Health and hygiene.   I. Title.
   RA564.85.M55   1991
   610'.82 – dc20   91–22711 CIP

Typeset by Graphicraft Typesetters Ltd., Hong Kong
Printed in Great Britain by St Edmundsbury Press Limited
Bury St Edmunds, Suffolk

Contents

Dedicated to my husband Bob
and to my granddaughter Esther

Preface

In conversation one day with my granddaughter, not then five years of age, she began to speculate, as children will, on what she might be when she grew up. I ventured the suggestion that she could become a doctor. 'Don't be silly' she said scornfully, 'girls can't be doctors.' This true anecdote shows just how soon the child is socialized into acceptance of what is and what is not appropriate to one of its gender. My granddaughter would have reacted similarly to a suggestion that she might be a bank manager, an engineer or a bus driver while a boy of like age would, I imagine, have treated with equal scorn a proposal that he might eventually take up nursing.

As the child, so the adult. The patient expects to meet male doctors, surgeons and gynaecologists, just as the nurse and the health visitor are expected to be female. Nevertheless, there is now a growing number of women doctors and a section of this book deals with their experiences, *vis-à-vis* their male colleagues, in medical school and in subsequent practice.

Studies of women have greatly expanded in recent years and within that wider framework the subject of women and health has received much attention; women, that is, not only as providers of health care but as recipients of it. Many research programmes have been undertaken regarding the health-related problems of women, the care received by them in various structures of the health services and the situation of female doctors, nurses, health scientists, and manual workers in hospitals. Research has been carried out by medical scientists, psychologists, sociologists, historians and others, each pursuing one or other interest from the standpoint of a particular discipline, some taking a feminist stance, others eschewing feminism. The results have been written up in a wide variety of learned journals or as separate publications, and to these writings must be added the range of statistical information emanating from the United States of America and the countries of the European Community.

Not surprisingly, this abundance of data tends to confusion and those who seek systematically to study the relationship of women to health and health care can find it difficult to know where to start and how to organize the large and diverse amount of material available. The intention of this book is to acquaint those who embark on such a project with at least some of the arguments, problems and research findings, in a way that is compact and comprehensible, so that it may be of use as a basis for further study. It is meant for those who are studying to become, or are already, health professionals, for students in social sciences, and for the participants of courses in women's studies.

The topics which could be included in an introductory volume such as this are numerous and selection was inevitable. Those chosen reflect my personal interests and those of many of my students, past and present. During the 1980s my students became increasingly interested in gender issues within the sociology of health and illness courses that I teach and I am indebted to them for their enthusiasm and intelligent interest. Truly can I say that while teaching them, I have been taught.

The following chapters are designed to be read independently of each other although it is hoped that they form a cohesive whole. The literature referred to and listed in the bibliography would be useful for further reading. The assumption throughout has been that readers will have an interest in the experiences of women as providers and users of health services.

This book is written for students of today. I hope that by the time my small granddaughter becomes a university student, at least some of the discussions and arguments concerning women's position in the social structure, will be outmoded.

1 Patterns of ill health in women

Women and men inhabit the same world but the world of women is different from that of men. Women live longer but suffer from more health problems during their lifetime and many of these problems are specific to the female gender. Patterns of ill health provide the framework within which people think about health problems and women, especially, make decisions regarding the health-related concerns of themselves and their families (the subject of Chapters 2, 3 and 4). It is within this framework that the health-care arrangements of society are formulated and health professionals are trained and operate (Chapters 5 and 6). This chapter focuses on gender differences in the nature and prevalence of disease and illness and on the difficulties which confront those who study them: it looks also at some of the important influences on patterns of ill health in women, such as social class, marital status and employment. Lastly, it will consider women's cigarette smoking and alcohol consumption, with which much ill health has been found to be associated.

Patterns of ill health

Studying diseases

It has been said that there are but two certainties in life – death and taxes. One is tempted to add a third – disease – since it is a rare human being who goes through life without suffering from any of the ills which afflict our species.

Registration of death is compulsory in advanced societies and a death certificate will include, with other information, the sex, age and occupation of the deceased and the cause of death. The last named is entered by a doctor and is later coded according to the International Classification of Diseases, Injuries and Causes of Death (ICD). A well-tried approach to the study of disease patterns is through the examination of trends in mortality and the ICD provides a useful, if imprecise, tool for this purpose. Imprecision arises from a number of causes: the doctor's task it not always easy; a bullet through the heart is conclusive enough but old people can suffer from various degenerative changes and the doctor may need to make a judgement as to the actual cause of death. Studies indicate that the cause (or causes) shown on a death certificate can conflict with hospital case notes and that post-mortem examination can reveal the presence of a disease of which the doctor who treated the patient was unaware. Coding causes of death also involves a judgement; the coder is required to allocate a specific ICD number to the information on the death certificate; coding practices differ from one country to another (Tuckett, 1976; Barker and Rose, 1984; Open University, 1985). Nevertheless, the attraction of using mortality statistics as indicators of disease patterns is that such statistics are routinely compiled and are based on statutory declarations.

Mortality figures indicate patterns of diseases which lead to death; they do not show how long the disease had been present before death, nor are they concerned with patterns of ill health which do not result in death. Minor ailments abound and there are major diseases which can be prevalent in a population yet seldom result in death. An example of the latter is osteoporosis, a disease experienced by many middle-aged and elderly persons, especially women, which involves the loss of bone mass and increases the danger of fractures. It is estimated that one woman in four will suffer the effects of osteoporosis but mortality statistics reflect only a very small number of deaths from this cause (Office of Health Economics, 1987). But death from 'complications' following a fracture, caused by a fall, due to osteoporosis, is something else and constitutes a good example of the difficulty in determining causes of death. For the purposes of analysing mortality patterns, however, the immediate cause, as recorded on the death certificate, is taken as the cause of death, but it is as well to bear in mind that causal factors are possibly wide ranging.

Despite the difficulties, it is easier to study patterns of death than it is to find out about patterns of ill health or 'morbidity' although some statistics are routinely collected. In Britain, the Hospital In-patient Enquiry records information on one in every ten hospital admissions, while the Royal College of General Practitioners collects data on patient consultations from a sample of its members. These methods are not without problems either. Perforce, the Hospital Enquiry can provide information only on in-patients but admission to hospital is often determined by social factors, e.g. care at home and the availability of hospital beds. Hospital statistics usually refer to disease episodes, not to patients, so that the admission of one patient five times, on each occasion with the same condition, is not differentiated from the admission of five separate individuals in a similar state of ill health. There are many people who would not trouble either the hospital or the general practitioner with a common cold (which might be influenza) or with a rash (which might be due to food poisoning) or even with a pain in the chest, which they will ascribe to indigestion, although a doctor might suspect heart trouble. One could cite many other instances of this sort of behaviour but the point is that hospital and general practitioner records do not tell the whole story.

Screening programmes are one way round the difficulty. Medical tests can be carried out on a defined population, e.g. schoolchildren, workers in a factory, even the residents of a town, in order to establish disease patterns, but the cost of such programmes is a deterrent and their routine use tends to be restricted to 'at risk' groups.

Another approach to the study of morbidity is to select a sample of the population and ask them about their health and their illnesses, either routinely at regular intervals (in Britain, the General Household Survey is the main example) or as a single research enquiry. Self-reported information of this kind poses problems of interpretation as respondents will vary in their knowledge of the nature and the severity of their own diseases. Not all respondents will be willing to report their health problems unreservedly (male respondents of a recent research found it more difficult to talk about emotional problems (neurosis) than did the women (Miles, 1988). People differ in their perceptions of what constitutes health and illness and their perceptions shape their answers. Even so, self-reporting provides much information on health and ill health which cannot be obtained in any other way (Blaxter, 1985; Blaxter, 1987a). Furthermore, it adds the dimension of personal experience to the body of information on morbidity.

Sociologists usually make a distinction between disease and illness. The term *disease*, in sociological literature, refers to a biological or clinically identified abnormality which is considered 'pathological' by medical practitioners; *illness* refers to a person's experience of being unwell. In such sense, disease is an 'objective' disorder, that is, assessed by someone other than the patient and illness is a 'subjective' feeling of symptoms, self-assessed by the individual (Helman, 1981; Armstrong, 1989). There is a third dimension of ill-health, i.e. the social and functional consequences which may follow disease or illness, and this is usually distinguished by the term *sickness*.

It is possible to have a disease without feeling ill. Someone may have diabetes without being aware of symptoms, and yet this condition might cause blindness in the not-too-distant future; another person, although aware of signs and symptoms e.g. teeth decay or a persistent cough, would assume them to be part of ordinary life or of 'getting older' (Tuckett, 1976; Miles, 1978; Armstrong, 1989), not as indications of illness. Conversely, it is possible to feel very unwell without the presence of a disease; pregnant women and teething infants are examples. The General Household Survey shows much reported illness co-existing with positive evaluations of general health; in fact the association between self-reported symptoms and self-assessment of overall health is somewhat slender (Macintyre, 1986).

The social role called 'sickness' might or might not accompany disease or illness and this will be explored in Chapter 3.

Gender differences in mortality

Medical statisticians usually examine rates of deaths rather than absolute numbers of deaths because the latter statistic is of limited use for comparisons of populations of varying size. (For explanations of the use of medical statistics, see Smith, 1968, and Open University, 1985.) Various rates are used: the *crude death rate* (CDR) in a particular year (per 1000 population) can be calculated according to a simple formula:

$$CDR = \frac{\text{Number of deaths that year}}{\text{Total population that year}} \times 1000$$

This rate, however, is affected by the age and sex of the total population and it is usual for age-specific death rates to be calculated for each sex. It is customary also to work with the *standardized mortality rate* (SMR) when a summary of the total population is needed; this is a method of comparing death rates between different sections of the population, holding other variables constant.

Since the beginning of the twentieth century, mortality rates for both women and men have fallen in Western industrial countries, but the reduction has been greater for women. Sex difference in mortality exists even before birth: male foetuses are more likely to be spontaneously aborted and stillbirth rates are higher among males. In adults, the higher level of male deaths persists in every age group, (Macfarlane and Mugford, 1984; Hart, 1988) and this pattern has been noted in most contemporary societies (Verbrugge, 1976, 1982; Nathanson, 1977; Waldron, 1982a, 1983a).

Trends in this century indicate that the difference between male and female death rates in early life has been declining, whereas in adults

Table 1.1 Expectation of life at birth, 1 year, 15, 45 and 65 years according to gender. Data for England & Wales, 1901–10 to 1983–85

	Birth		1 year		15 years		45 years		65 years	
Year	M	F	M	F	M	F	M	F	M	F
1901–10	48.5	52.4	55.7	58.3	47.3	50.1	22.3	25.5	10.8	12.0
1910–12	51.5	55.4	57.5	60.3	48.6	51.4	23.9	26.3	11.0	12.4
1930–32	58.7	62.9	62.3	65.5	51.2	54.3	25.5	28.3	11.3	13.1
1950–52	66.4	71.5	67.7	72.4	54.4	59.0	26.5	30.8	11.7	14.3
1970–72	69.0	75.3	69.4	75.4	55.8	61.8	27.4	32.9	12.2	16.1
1980–82	71.1	77.1	71.0	76.9	57.3	63.1	28.7	34.1	13.1	17.1
1983–85	71.8	77.7	71.6	77.4	57.9	63.6	29.2	34.5	13.4	17.5

Source: OPCS, quoted by Office of Health Economics, 1987.

the difference has grown greater (Macfarlane and Mugford, 1984; Hart, 1988).

An alternative way of looking at mortality is to calculate *life expectancy*: estimates in Britain show that girls born in 1983–85 can expect to live about six years (5.9) longer than boys born in the same year, to 77.7 years and 71.8 years, respectively (Table 1.1). In the United States the difference in life expectancy is greater: at the end of 1970, an almost eight-year intergender difference was noted (Verbrugge, 1981).

According to historians, the current lower mortality rate for women is a relatively recent phenomenon and in the past men outlived women. Edward Shorter (1984) quotes evidence according to which in prehistoric times the expectation of life for males was longer by about 20 per cent and goes on to point out that village studies conducted by historical demographers show consistent female excess mortality prior to the mid-nineteenth century. Only at the end of the nineteenth century did the present pattern of women's longer life expectancy become established.

Shorter attributes women's comparatively higher mortality rates in past societies to the particularly harsh conditions of their lives (Shorter, 1984, p. 237):

Women were more liable than men to die at certain ages because their lives at those ages were much harder than men's, and their resistance to infection was lower. Two circumstances in particular emerge: the grinding routine of field work in rural areas, and the rigours of married life.

Higher female mortality rates continue to prevail in some contemporary societies where industrialization is less than in Western countries (Waldron, 1982a, 1983b). For example, in Bangladesh, India, Nepal and Papua New Guinea men have the greater life expectancy. Women in these lands experience harsh working conditions and frequent pregnancies which together with a comparatively low level of obstetric care leads to high maternal mortality (Waldron, 1983b; United Nations, 1981). Thus gender differences in life expectancy are closely connected with levels of economic development. Indeed, examining international trends, researchers argue that the longer the life expectancy of a given population, the greater the increase in the life expectancy of females and the wider the intergender difference in life expectancy (Leviathan and Cohen, 1985).

As mentioned above, medical practitioners are obliged to record the 'cause of death' on death certificates. Examination of the data thus obtained reveals quite significant differences in the causes of death of men and of women. For example, in Britain, for young adults under the age of 35, accidents and violence account for 70 per cent of male deaths as against 35 per cent of female deaths (Central Statistical Office, 1986). In the United States, for the 25–44 age group, accidents are the main cause of death for men but for women, malignant neoplasms rank first with accidents second, whereas for people aged 45–64, heart diseases take over as the main killers of men with malignant neoplasms remaining as the main cause of female death (Verbrugge, 1986). Once over 65, heart diseases overwhelmingly appear as the principal cause of death for people of both sexes, although it needs to be borne in mind that the term refers to a group of diseases rather than a single cause.

Statistics of mortality in females show coronary heart disease to be a significant cause of death, an interesting finding because until recently research on this disease, especially the possible connection between personality and vulnerability to it, focused on males. While it is true that there are more male than female deaths from this cause, coronary heart disease is an important cause of premature death in women. Also, in Britain, between the years 1978 and 1986, the reduction in male deaths from this cause was more than double that for females (perhaps because medical research concentrated on males) (Office of Health Economics, 1987, p. 28).

Table 1.2 shows the six main causes of female mortality in England & Wales. For women under 65, breast cancer is the second highest cause of death and the outlook can only be described as gloomy. Trends indicate an increasing mortality from this disease in older age groups (over 54) while improvement among younger age groups is at best marginal, or non-existent (Office of Health Economics, 1987, p. 31).

Table 1.2 The six principal causes of mortality for females under 75 years and their significance in the 0–64 and 75 and over age groupings (England & Wales, 1986), expressed as total numbers (*n*) and percentages of total number

Disease	Under 65		Under 75		75 and over	
	n	Percen-tage	*n*	Percen-tage	*n*	Percen-tage
Coronary heart disease	6690	15.2	23085	22.7	46509	24.5
Cerebrovascular disease	2844	6.5	10008	9.8	34218	18.0
Breast cancer	5542	12.6	8889	8.7	4752	2.5
Lung cancer	2981	6.8	6723	6.6	3299	1.7
Cancer of Genito-urinary organs	3617	8.2	6485	6.4	3706	2.0
Cancer of digestive organs and peritoneum	3628	8.3	8677	8.5	10462	5.5
Totals	25302	57.6	63867	62.7	102946	54.2

Source: *OPCS Monitor*, quoted by Office of Health Economics, 1987.

Gender differences in morbidity

It was pointed out at the beginning of this chapter that the examination of recorded causes of death and of the prevalence of medically-diagnosed diseases among the population provides only a partial picture of overall ill health. Another important dimension is the subjective experience of illness: it is consistently found that women report more illnesses than do men.

In Britain, the Nottingham Health Profile showed the self-assessed health of women to be significantly worse than that of men (Hunt *et al.*, 1985); a similar finding was made by Blaxter (1985). In *The Health and Life-style Survey* (Cox *et al.*, 1987) respondents were given a symptoms checklist and 'illness scores' were calculated by the number of reported symptoms (Table 1.3). As elsewhere, the results showed that women reported higher rates of illness than men at all ages. There could be a difference in reporting but it is possible that women typically experience more discomfort and pain of a non-life-threatening kind.

The particular health problems that people in Britain take to their doctors are indicated by the survey of the Royal College of General Practitioners; Table 1.4 shows the categories of diseases which most

Table 1.3 Illness scores based on the reported occurrence of symptoms: percentage declaring high rates

Age group	Males	Females
18–39	12.3	21.8
40–59	16.8	31.1
60+	21.5	32.4

Source: Blaxter, 1987a, p. 12.

frequently prompt patients to consult their general practitioners. The highest consultation rates are for respiratory disorders of various kinds and although there is no great difference between women and men in this respect, more women consult their doctors with such problems. The difference in consultation rates for cystitis and urinary problems is understandably sex-related, and the difference in hypertension may be partly due to the fact that the blood pressure of women is more frequently taken, this test being routinely associated with antenatal care and prescriptions for oral contraceptives and hormone-replacement therapy.

Some of the most striking gender differences occur in consultations for psychiatric symptoms (depression and anxiety) and this will be

Table 1.4 Patients consulting general practitioners for selected diseases. Rates per 1000 at risk

Disease	Females	Males
Upper respiratory tract infection (non-febrile)	99.7	82.7
Acute bronchitis	58.4	57.8
Acute tonsilitis	45.6	38.5
Upper respiratory tract infection (febrile)	43.9	43.3
Uncomplicated hypertension	42.7	31.4
Cystitis and urinary infection	39.0	7.9
Depressive disorder	38.3	12.4
Anxiety disorder/state	37.6	16.0
Abdominal pain	36.3	22.7
Intestinal disease	34.0	32.4
Conjunctivitis	32.3	24.1
Osteoarthritis	31.8	14.4

Source: Royal College of General Practitioners, 1986.

Table 1.5 Consultation rates per 1000 population for symptoms, signs and ill-defined conditions, based on age group

Gender	15–24	25–44	45–64	65–74	All
Female	174.0	165.5	160.6	196.8	182.4
Male	91.5	99.5	119.6	159.9	134.4

Source: Office of Health Economics, 1987.

discussed separately. It is also important to note that the same survey (Royal College of General Practitioners, 1986) showed that women consult their doctors much more often than do men, with a range of problems, classified by the International Classification of Diseases as 'symptoms, signs and ill-defined conditions', which includes headaches, dizziness, chest-pains, fatigue, tiredness, nausea, skin eruptions, etc.; the difference is especially marked in the younger age groups (see Table 1.5).

In the United States, Lois Verbrugge examined the National Health Interview Survey and the National Ambulatory Medical Care Survey which she used, together with data from hospital and community statistics, to compile an illness profile of American men and women of different age groups (Verbrugge, 1986). Her findings were similar to the British data. For younger adults of both sexes, the principal daily health problems were respiratory ailments while for the middle-aged, musculo-skeletal problems dominated: the latter domination was even more pronounced for older adults of both sexes. Verbrugge noted that women experienced more daily symptoms and higher rates of all types of acute conditions (except injuries at younger ages) and more hospital stays. It is interesting to note that these imbalances persisted even when consultations for reproductive disorders and events were discounted.

Explanations of gender differences in mortality
and morbidity

According to Macintyre (1986, p. 395):

Differences between the sexes appear to be sufficiently obvious for most social and health data to be presented and analysed separately for each sex. The assumption that there will be distinctive profiles for each sex on any given variable is so taken-for-granted, however, that the data often remain treated separately rather than being subject to systematic comparison or attempts to account for the difference. In this sense, as Morgan [Morgan, 1980] has argued: 'Gender, as a key variable, is both ubiquitous and hidden'.

How can differences in mortality and morbidity patterns between women and men be explained? Uncertainties and controversies surround the subject of gender differences in health and disease patterns. Understanding why these differences exist is crucial, however, both for increasing knowledge of underlying social processes and for the practical purpose of improving the health of the population. At a general level there are three possible ways of accounting for these gender differences, namely the *'artefact'*, the *genetic* and the *social* causation explanations. These explanations, which are not mutually exclusive, have been much debated.

The possibility that differences in the morbidity statistics for women and men are due to an 'artefact' has been considered by a number of researchers (Gove, 1978, 1984; Waldron, 1983a; Macintyre, 1986; Whitehead, 1988). According to this explanation, differences are apparent rather than real, the supposition being that while women's health is no worse than men's they are more inclined to take notice of symptoms and are readier to consult doctors and to undergo treatment. It is also possible that women are more willing to co-operate in health surveys. (Differences in the perceptions and in the behaviour of women and men with regard to their respective health problems will be explored in the following three chapters.) That doctors' diagnoses may be influenced by the sex of their patients, and the like possibility that their recording of the causes of death may be influenced by the sex of the deceased, are other 'artefacts' which could tend to gender differences.

According to the second, genetic, explanation, gender differences in patterns of mortality and morbidity are influenced by a range of genetic factors and by a complex interaction between environment and heredity. The rather controversial evidence was reviewed by Ingrid Waldron (1982a,b, 1983a): genetic factors certainly appear to contribute to differential patterns but do not on their own provide a satisfactory explanation. Thus, for example, differences in reproductive anatomy and physiology have an important bearing on mortality and on disease patterns, women having more complex and more demanding reproductive functions. Women may be endowed with greater resistance to infectious diseases due to genes carried by the X chromosome that influence immune functioning; endogenous female sex hormones may reduce women's risk of ischaemic heart disease (Waldron, 1976, 1983a). Genetic and environmental factors interact in many ways: Waldron argued that a given genetic factor has variable effects on mortality differences depending on environmental conditions, such as the availability of obstetric services (Waldron, 1983b). For example, males seem to have a genetically greater vulnerability to foetal mortality, but this mortality has been much reduced in developed industrial countries with improved maternal health and obstetric skills (Hart, 1988).

The third general explanation lies in the social causation hypothesis which argues that certain aspects of women's and men's lives render them more, or less, vulnerable to certain diseases and that different kinds of lives lead, in complex ways, to different patterns of mortality and morbidity. It is suggested that women's lower death rates are partly due to their being less likely than men to take risks, i.e. less likely to act in ways which can lead to accidents and violence. As already shown, among young adults, male mortality from such causes much exceeds that of women. Studies of children's games show that boys play in riskier ways and meet with more accidents than do girls (Ginsburg and Miller, 1982). Boys are socialized from an early age to value 'toughness' and 'courage', and girls to display timidity and gentleness. Boys are allowed more freedom to play away from the home, while girls are encouraged to remain in the home or its immediate vicinity. Patterns of differential risk taking continue into adulthood, when men incur more accidents of various kinds than do women. In the United States, accidental drownings and fatal accidents involving guns are five times higher for males than females (Waldron, 1983b). Men drive faster and with less care than women, and violate traffic rules more frequently, factors which may well be the major cause of higher rates of fatal motor accidents among men (Veevers, 1982). There are gender differences in smoking and in the partaking of alcohol and drugs, men in each case being the more likely to indulge in these practices, confirmatory evidence of their greater risk taking. These differences constitute an important aspect of disease patterns.

An interesting research, carried out by Leviathan and Cohen (1985), may serve to illuminate the issues under discussion. Their research was conducted in Israel among kibbutz society where the lives of women and men are more similar than is usually the case in Westernized societies. All adults are engaged full time in work outside their homes. There is no compulsory retirement, all continuing to labour, on a modified basis where necessary, up to the age of 80 and even beyond. Adults of both sexes experience the same economic pressures and responsibilities and equally participate in family roles and community life; their daily schedules and routines are alike and they enjoy similar and potential social support. Moreover, those who are born on a kibbutz have similar experiences of schooling and military service. When the researchers examined mortality figures and calculated gender differences in life expectancy, they found the latter to be greatly reduced, the intergender difference being almost three years less in the kibbutz population than was to be expected from calculations based on figures for the general population of the country. (The expected difference was 7.1 years; the actual was 4.5 years.) According to Leviathan and Cohen, the reduction of the gender difference was due pre-eminently to the greater similarity of life-experiences and social roles of women and men *vis-à-vis* non-kibbutz society. However, (Leviathan and Cohen, 1985, p. 550) point out that they are

> in no position to claim that biological and genetic factors are not important. Even in the current kibbutz population we still find intergender differences that could be related either to the remainder of the differentiated gender roles on the kibbutz or to some biological factors.

Influences on women's health

Social class

Not all of the women in a given society (nor all of the men for that matter) experience the same degree of ill health: social class, employment, ethnic origin and marital status greatly influence the extent and the nature of morbidity.

Social scientists and health professionals in Britain have for a considerable time been paying attention to class inequalities in health. In recent years, several major reports have highlighted the correlation between health and social position (Townsend and Davidson, 1982; Whitehead, 1988) yet, although the existence of this correlation has been known for over a century, each fresh evidence of it seems to occasion surprise. To aver that there is a lineal connection between poverty, poor living conditions and ill health might be thought to do no more than state the obvious; it could be, however, that the modern welfare state has created an expectation that earlier disparities in sickness rates between the poor and the better off have been eliminated, so that evidence of their continuing presence is both unwelcome and surprising to many people. According to Blaxter (Blaxter, 1981, p. 219):

> A great deal of effort has gone into the task of proving again and again, that (these) socially associated differences in the health status of children do exist: almost as if this were something society did not wish to believe, and had to re-discover at regular intervals.

To quote another social scientist (Macintyre, 1986, p. 393):

While it has been observed for some time that a person's social class of origin or achievement, gender, marital status, age, ethnic group and area of residence, are all correlated with his or her mental and physical health and likelihood of death (from all causes or specific causes), detailed study of why this should be so is surprisingly sparse. Indeed, the existence of the correlations themselves, which would not have surprised observers in the nineteenth century, is often treated as if it were a novel disclosure.

Researchers employ a range of indicators of social class position and have demonstrated their correlation with the health of the population. Table 1.6 shows the relationship between certain of these indicators and the death ratios of women of various ages.

Another illustration of the association between social class differences and women's mortality rates (also based on SMR) is the following: among single women in Britain, those with non-manual jobs and a car had an SMR of 69; those with manual jobs and no car had an SMR of 178. Among married housewives, for those with husbands in a non-manual occupation, with a car and living in owner-occupied housing, the SMR was 65; for those with husbands in manual occupations, no car and living in rented housing, the SMR was 161 (Whitehead, 1988, p. 238).

Indicators such as house ownership, access to a car and educational attainments may have a direct link with health status: for example,

Table 1.6 Mortality in England & Wales 1971–81: women aged 15–59 at death

Socio-economic indicators	Standardized mortality ratios
Housing tenure	
Owner-occupied	83
Privately rented	106
Local authority	117
Education	
Degree	66
Non-degree higher qualification	78
A levels only	80
None or not stated	102
Access to cars	
One or more cars	83
No access to a car	135

Source: Whitehead, 1988, p. 237.

those without cars would find it more difficult to attend surgeries; those living in crowded or poor conditions would be more exposed to infections; a lower educational level would probably mean a lower level of health knowledge. But such indicators also show the general association between level of health and social position: low wages, rented housing, lower education and many other features of low socioeconomic status correlate with poor health. The perceptions and actions of women vary according to their position in the social structure and such variations will be discussed in subsequent chapters.

Work

Some people thrive on work; for others, it is at best a necessary evil. Its opposite, unemployment, can be seen as a challenge or a disaster.

Although paid labour may be viewed as beneficial, numerous investigations have demonstrated that employment-related stress can harm both the physical and the mental well-being of workers (Brenner and Mooney, 1983; Cherry, 1984a,b; O'Brien, 1984; Caplan *et al.*, 1985) and studies of occupational hazards have shown that specific work environments and tasks may be injurious to the health of employees (Fox and Goldblatt, 1982; Chavkin, 1984). Lack of paid work, or unemployment, can also be damaging to health: in recent decades, an increasing volume of research evidence has drawn attention to the numerous physical and emotional health problems that can be attributed to loss of work or failure to obtain it (for a review of the literature see Warr, 1987).

Ill health can be a cause as well as a consequence of not working: studies of people suffering from chronic sickness, and other disabling conditions, have shown that job problems and unemployment are typically experienced by them (Blaxter, 1976; Anderson and Bury, 1988).

Within the wider complexities of the work–health relationship there lies the special issue of women and domestic work. Women, no less than men, can experience health problems related to paid employment, or the lack of it, but for them, or at least very many of them, there are, in addition, the constant demands of unwaged domestic work and childcare with their attendant health implications.

In contemporary Western societies, considerable emphasis is placed on the moral value of work both for the individual and for the community. For adult males, this usually means a single paid job at any one time and the socially most acceptable way of life for them is to be in employment, without interruption, between the completion of their education and retirement. Women also are expected to enter the labour market when their formal education is finished but it is entirely acceptable that they should leave their jobs, periodically, or even permanently, in order to devote their time to childcare and domestic work. In the second half of the twentieth century, the proportion of women in the labour force of many countries has increased (a feature of this increase has been the growing tendency for mothers of children to return to employment); for example, in the United States, the proportion of women in the labour force in 1949, 25 per cent, had increased to 43 per cent by 1982. The parallel figures for the United Kingdom were 31 and 39 per cent and for Australia 22 and 37 per cent. Current figures for (West) Germany and Japan indicate the same trend (U.S. Department of Labor, 1977; Organization for Economic Co-operation and Development, 1985).

A large proportion of married women in the United States and Britain have paid employment (Martin and Roberts, 1984). Nevertheless, these women continue to work in the home, domestic tasks, child rearing and caring for disabled and frail elderly family members being regarded essentially as the duty of women. How does work, paid or unpaid, or the want of it, affect the health of women?

Paid employment and domestic work

The increase in the number of women, especially married women, in paid employment has led to researchers investigating the relationship between women's health and employment status: is it more beneficial for women's health for them to be engaged solely on domestic work in the home, or to combine it with paid employment outside the home? Underlying these studies of employment status and health is the assumption that the main burden of domestic work and childcare falls on women, whether they have outside employment or not (a correct assumption, as research on the domestic division of labour indicates, see Land, 1981; Graham, 1984) and that women have the choice of undertaking paid employment or of not doing so. Surveys on employment status and health are bedevilled by methodological problems and suffer also from lack of conceptual clarity. Concepts of work and health are ambiguous, besides which surveys have often neglected to differentiate between types of employment and between women with varying domestic roles. (For a review of methodological problems, see Clarke, 1983.) However, some general findings are interesting and point the way to future research.

It is a consistent research finding that housewives have more health problems than are experienced by women with paid jobs outside the home (Gove and Tudor, 1973; Welch and Booth, 1977; Warr and Parry, 1982). An examination of data from the Health Interview Survey of the United States revealed that housewives evaluated their own health less positively than did women and men in paid employment (Table 1.7).

Table 1.7 Perceived health status of housewives, employed women and employed men, aged 45–64. Percentage assessed health as 'excellent'

Employed men	38.1
Employed women	38.7
Housewives	27.6

Source: Nathanson, 1980, p. 465.

Examining another of the indicators used by researchers, the relationship between employment status and mortality, Passannante and Nathanson (1985) studied death certificates in Wisconsin, and found that housewives experienced considerable disadvantage: for younger and middle-aged women (16–44, 45–54 and 55–59) the death rate of housewives was approximately twice as high as that of employed women (Table 1.8)

There are a number of reasons why paid employment outside the home can be thought beneficial for women's health, among them self-esteem and a sense of accomplishment. Such work is a socially-valued activity; domestic work, by contrast, is socially devalued, especially when it embraces no element of childcare. A personal sense of worth is an important constituent of well-being and one that is more likely to be attained by women with paid employment and its concomitant financial independence and wider social contacts, than by women who are constrained by housework and feelings of financial dependence and powerlessness (Chesler, 1972). However, while such arguments hold true for very many women, they are by no means applicable to them all.

The values attached to paid employment differ across social class categories and ethnic and other affiliations, and are influenced by the nature and the setting thereof. The executive office and the factory floor are much more than just alternative workplaces; the nurse enjoys

Table 1.8 Age-specific death rates (per 1000) of housewives and the female experienced labour force in Wisconsin, 1974–78

Age	Housewives	Labour force
16–44	1.15	0.51
45–54	5.44	2.33
55–59	8.44	4.73
60–64	10.96	10.12

Source: Passannante and Nathanson, 1985.

a prestige not accorded to the woman who cleans the hospital; a woman's age and the situation of her children (if any) will affect attitudes to her working. Paid employment itself would hardly be countenanced in certain circles which would nevertheless regard charitable work as entirely acceptable.

Arguments have been adduced according to which paid employment might damage, rather than benefit, the health of some women. The domestic division of labour is unequal, with husbands doing less work in the home than their wives, with the consequence that the wife with outside employment finds herself doing two jobs, both of them occupying many hours of the day (Oakley, 1974; Martin and Roberts, 1984; Sharpe, 1984). The resultant overwork leads to fatigue and exhaustion and, in return, to higher levels of morbidity. The woman in this situation is also liable to the strains and stresses attendant upon the dilemma of trying to serve two masters, of constantly having to choose whether to put first the needs of the employer or the family. A growing body of research evidence points to the physical and psychological symptoms experienced by mothers of young children endeavouring to combine the responsibilities of home and workplace (Gove and Hughes, 1979: Shimmin *et al.*, 1981; Cleary and Mechanic, 1983).

Further support for the proposition that outside employment can be damaging to women is to be found in the consistently higher male mortality rates, the suggestion here being that because many women are not exposed to the alleged harmful influences of the work setting, the mortality rates of women generally are thereby improved. Those who argue that paid employment is harmful to the health of women distrust statistics which indicate the relatively poorer health of housewives without paid employment, pointing out that women suffering from chronic sickness or disability and consequently being unemployable, prefer to describe themselves as 'housewives' rather than as 'chronic-sick unemployed'. Thus, figures based on large surveys are distorted: instead of comparing initially healthy female populations and seeing whether employment or domestic work is more conducive to good health, they compare a healthy female workforce with women, a proportion of whom are chronically sick.

The arguments for and against the outside employment of women are less contradictory than might at first appear. More detailed studies of women of different ages and of diverse family backgrounds provide evidence of the kinds of women who benefit, and those who do not benefit, from such employment.

The study of Constance Nathanson, in the United States, showed that employment is most beneficial for the health of those women who lack home-centred social support and who most need to find a sense of accomplishment and personal worth, lacking in their roles as house-wives (Nathanson, 1980, p. 470):

> Not only is employment positively associated with perceived health status, but the association is most marked among women with the least access to opportunities for self-esteem and social support alternative to employment.

This is also consistent with the findings of the London-based study of depression in women, where it was noted that vulnerability was increased amongst women without close, intimate and confiding relationships (Brown and Harris, 1978). In this study, too, employment outside the home was found to be beneficial in that it reduced women's vulnerability to depression.

An interesting comparative study on this subject was carried out in Finland by Elina Haavio-Mannila (1986) who examined statistics from four countries (Denmark, Finland, Norway and Sweden). She looked at patterns of morbidity of husbands and wives in households where the wives worked in paid employment and where they did not. In addition to overall morbidity, she examined the level of 'anxiety-symptoms', arguing that this provides a good indicator of stress consequent upon too many demands and conflicting obligations: Table 1.9 summarizes her findings. Inequalities in morbidity are much greater in families where wives stay at home than in families where they work outside the home, wives in the latter being healthier. The author attributes this to the beneficial effects of paid work on women's health and also to the higher income level of these families. Anxiety levels are relatively high amongst women with paid employment (except in Sweden) an indication of the strains experienced by women endeavouring to fulfil two, often contradictory, roles. Haavio-Mannila in an earlier study showed that women in Helsinki were drawn two ways: employed mothers expressed more happiness, more satisfaction with life, but also had higher anxiety rates than did mothers without paid employment (Haavio-Mannila, 1979). Apparently, the reward of employment was lower morbidity; the cost, a higher anxiety level.

The picture is more complex, however: social class and the types of occupation that women engage in, greatly influence morbidity. Nathanson (1980) noted that women with relatively low educational attainments ('less than high school education') were much more likely than the better educated to benefit from employment, taking the view that such women had small opportunity to find self-esteem and worth in unwaged domestic work. Brown and Harris (1978) also found that it was the working-class women, with young children at home, who were most vulnerable to depression and who most needed outside employment to boost their self-confidence: working-class women ben-

Table 1.9 Morbidity and symptoms of anxiety of husbands and wives in families with wife at home and wife in paid employment in Scandinavia in 1972 (percentages)

Morbidity/anxiety	Denmark	Finland	Norway	Sweden
Morbidity				
Wife at home				
Husbands	15	27	15	16
Wives	24	38	22	24
Sex ratio (F/M)	160	141	147	150
Wife working for pay				
Husbands	15	27	18	15
Wives	16	31	20	16
Sex ratio (F/M)	107	115	111	107
Symptoms of anxiety				
Wife at home				
Husbands	52	68	48	46
Wives	62	68	61	57
Sex ratio (F/M)	119	100	127	124
Wife working for pay				
Husbands	50	63	46	44
Wives	64	72	69	47
Sex ratio (F/M)	128	114	150	107

Source: Haavio-Mannila, 1985.

efited from employment more than did middle-class women. Indeed, it can be argued that work outside the home is most beneficial for the health of those women whose home environment is adverse with poor housing, no access to resources such as car or telephone, and with financial hardship (Warr and Parry, 1982).

However, it also appears that working-class women who most need to get away from home for their mental well-being, and who are most in need of additional earnings, are very likely to find themselves working, at the workplace as well as in the home, in conditions tending to excessive fatigue. In a British study, Sara Arber and her colleagues examined the General Household Survey (an annual sample survey in which adults in 14 000 households are interviewed) and compared the self-reported ill health of employed women and of housewives (Arber *et al.*, 1985). They noted that women working in manual occupations (skilled and unskilled) or in low-level non-manual jobs and with dependent children (under 16 years) at home, reported considerably more ill health than did comparable housewives who remained at home. (The occupational class of housewives was based on their last employment.) Comparable women, whose jobs were managerial or professional (also with dependent children at home) reported much less illness. Arber and her colleagues argued that women in managerial and professional jobs have better financial resources which they can use to reduce the burden of homework and childcare, so alleviating fatigue and stress. They may also be better placed to control their work, with a measure of flexibility, thus better accommodating the demands of childcare, while women working in lower level employment are more likely to be tied to rigid work schedules (Arber *et al.*, 1985, p. 393).

The data gained by Arber *et al.* also showed that part-time work benefited working mothers more than did full-time work, and that such was the case for all occupational classes. This is understandable, as the authors themselves assert, because part-time workers are able to combine the best of both worlds, gaining self-esteem, wider social contacts and financial rewards from employment while avoiding at least some of the stress and over-work experienced by mothers working full time.

Merely to note that working-class women with full-time jobs outside the home, having also children to attend to and a house to run, experience stress, exhaustion and much ill health, says nothing about solutions. Overwork is the most obvious cause and can largely be attributed to inequality in the domestic division of labour; only where childcare and housework are evenly divided between wives and husbands can the health of such women be expected to improve.

Occupational hazards

Traditionally, research on occupational hazards and accidents has been centred on areas of employment having a predominantly male labour force. The employment conditions of women in mills and match factories now bear little resemblance to those of the early years of the industrial era. The hazardous occupations of mining, fishing and construction work today employ few women and it has come to be thought that women workers generally are less exposed to serious work-related hazards than are male workers.

However, recent research has indicated that industries employing a largely female labour force, and which were not previously thought of as particularly hazardous, none the less expose their employees to physical, chemical and biological risks. In addition, current medical views, linking stress to physical and mental illness, suggest that occupational stress potentially affects health. Large numbers of women work in stressful work settings, and this occupational hazard has received more attention in recent years (Stellman, 1978).

There are many health risks attaching to the 'new' industries. Baker and Woodrow (1984) writing about the electronics industry, point out that although it has been talked of as the 'clean', 'light', industry of the future, surveys show that it relies on the use of potentially dangerous substances and that few of the hundreds of different chemicals employed have been adequately tested for their safety. Moreover (Baker and Woodrow, 1984, p. 25):

Every step of the production process requires the use of these corrosive and toxic chemicals, often in combinations that are not found in other settings. Yet the scientific community has done very little to research the synergistic or combined, effects of these chemicals, and the state of the art is just not keeping pace with work-place realities. The technology changes at a lightning pace, as fierce competition within the industry dictates constant growth and innovation.

Women fill the majority of the industry's assembly jobs. In Silicon Valley, California, more than three-quarters of the production workers are women, many of Asian and Hispanic origin. In Third-World countries where the labour-intensive and low-skilled part of the production is concentrated the workforce is almost entirely female (Baker and Woodrow note that in South-East Asia, women make up 90 per cent of the electronics workforce).

Office work, where the proportion of female employees is high, has come under increasing scrutiny. In the United States, eight out of ten clerical workers are women; they work in modern offices, using word-processors, computers, photocopying machines, etc. It is widely assumed that offices provide clean and safe places of employment, but recent studies suggest that clerical workers may be exposed to hazardous methanol and ozone levels emanating from machines (Stellman, 1977) and that women operating office machines for many hours a day can be affected by musculo-skeletal pain in the back, neck and arms. Artificial lighting and ventilation also constitute hazards (Fleishman, 1984). Moreover, there has been growing concern over radiation emissions from video-display terminals (Henifin, 1984).

The employment of women in a variety of industries with a high risk of exposure to carcinogens is also an area of concern (Waldron, 1980). Certain risks are especially high for pregnant women: many functions of the body undergo marked changes in pregnancy (for example, the respiratory functions, fat storage, hormone production, etc.) and there is evidence that working in some hazardous environments poses an increased risk, not only to the pregnant woman, but to the foetus also (Chavkin, 1984).

Recent research has paid much attention to stress in the work environment of both men and women. Women entering the labour force become subject to the stresses that male workers are accustomed to, concerning working conditions, workloads and demands, career structure, competition, etc., all implying exposure to stress-related diseases (Cooper and Marshall, 1976; Davidson and Cooper, 1981). The discrimination and disadvantages experienced by women at work, add their own special sources of stress to those inherent in the job situation; see Spencer and Podmore (1987) on the experiences of women in the professions of medicine, law, politics, etc., and Chavkin (1984) regarding women in office and factory work. Stress-related diseases in women have been demonstrated by longitudinal investigations such as the Framingham Heart and Hypertension Study which indicated that a large proportion of women clerical workers are at risk of coronary heart disease (Haines and Feinleib, 1980).

In recent years much information has come to light about sexual harassment at the workplace, and it can be argued that the experience of this nuisance and even the apprehension of its occurrence, constitute a source of stress for women employees. Surveys suggest that a large proportion of women workers (50 to 70 per cent in some workplaces) report such harassment, often in the form of unwanted sexual advances and propositions followed by retaliation for non-cooperation (Gruber and Bjorn, 1982; Crull, 1982). Stress can lead to health problems, both physical and emotional, and in one study, over a third of the women who reported sexual harassment pointed to physical ailments which they thought had been brought about by it. Symptoms listed by these women included severe headaches, nausea, fatigue and vomiting (Crull, 1984).

Domestic work, no less than outside employment, is accompanied by health hazards, and women, who do the majority of household tasks, tend to be more at risk. Information concerning hazards in the home is often inadequate (Rosenberg, 1984):

> The experts' advice to women centers on the areas of housework, child-bearing and rearing. Books on these subjects are cheap, written in simple language, and readily available in supermarkets, drugstores and bookstores ... On the other hand, it is very difficult to find information about product or appliance safety. Women who do domestic labour are forced to rely on advertisers for information about the chemical content or safety aspects of their products.

Any view of the home as a safe place is belied by statistics which show that home accidents rank high among causes of accidental death. Coal fires, electric and paraffin heaters, all pose threats of burning as does cooking, hot water and so on. Glass and kitchen implements are responsible for often severe lacerations while very many cleaning agents carry warnings as to their possibly harmful effects. The list is long and the housewife has constantly to be on her guard. The more tired and overworked she is, the greater the danger.

Unemployment

Research on the consequences of unemployment has typically been carried out on men, while the subject of unemployed women has largely been neglected. Economic hardship was considered to be the most severe consequence of unemployment and men were (and frequently still are) regarded as the 'breadwinner'. Even when researchers started to interest themselves in other aspects of unemployment, the assumption was often made that men stood to be affected more than women who had alternative, acceptable social roles as wives, mothers or daughters, to fall back upon. Research on unemployed women is complicated by the difficulty of distinguishing between the 'unemployed' and the 'non-employed' – the former being those who are out of a job but wish to have and seek employment, the latter having no such wish (Warr, 1987). Indeed, clear distinctions are difficult, as between the unemployed and the non-employed, as defined; there are women who would like some paid employment provided that it could be fitted in with domestic responsibilities, mothers of young children being an obvious example. Studies of women who are clearly unemployed, as demonstrated by their registration with official agencies, show that they experience problems which are very similar to those of men in the same situation, their psychological and physical health and well-being tending to be affected (Verbrugge, 1983: Martin and Wallace, 1985; Warr, 1987). Being out of a job brings, beside economic anxieties, loss of structure to one's life and loss of self-respect. Unemployed people typically report depression, irritability, insomnia, and general nervousness. A British study on the consequences of factory closure reported more frequent medical consultations (both in general practice and in hospitals) – especially among women employees who had lost their jobs (Beale and Nethercott, 1985). In another study, women (particularly older women) typically reported that job loss led to isolation and loneliness (Martin and Wallace, 1985).

It also has to be noted that the health of married women can be affected by their husband's loss of employment: Cohrane and Stopes-Roe (1981) found high levels of depression and anxiety symptoms among wives of unemployed men.

Marital status

Durkheim, in 1897, suggested that the state of being unmarried impacts differently upon the well-being of men and of women, the former faring the worse (Durkheim, 1952). Evidence today shows that married people have lower death rates than the never-married, the divorced and the widowed, a finding which holds true for both sexes although the difference between the death rates of 'single' and married people is less for women than for men, at all ages. With regard to morbidity, married men report better health than do single men although no such difference is revealed in the case of women (Macintyre, 1986). Marriage, then, is beneficial to health, with men profiting most in that respect, a contention supported by the British *Health and Life-style Survey* which contrasted illness scores of people over 60, respectively living alone and with their spouses (Table 1.10). After all, this age category would include many long-married couples, well-attuned to each other and yet, among such, wives recorded the higher illness score. As opposed to people living alone, married men were markedly more healthy, married women only marginally so.

It is possible to speculate on the reasons for married people having lower illness rates, and for the health of wives appearing to benefit less than that of their husbands. It is likely that couples have a healthier diet than those who live alone, especially men who would not, in youth, have acquired domestic skills, and who may rely more on ready-made meals and fast foods. Spouses note symptoms of illness in each other which those living alone might miss or choose to ignore; since wives have prime responsibility for the health of the family, they are usually knowledgeable about health and thus are more likely to pick up symptoms in their husbands than vice-versa (Graham, 1984). The situation with home nursing is similar, with the sick wife likely to receive a lesser quality of care than will her husband in the reverse situation and with married people faring better than those living alone. Social support and involvement with the community have an im-

Table 1.10 Illness scores: comparison of different household circumstances for those aged 60 and over (expressed as percentage with high illness score)

	Living alone	Living with spouse
Males	33	24
Females	38	34

Source: Blaxter, 1987a, p. 13.

portant bearing on the health and well-being of individuals and it is
important to note here that the single, widowed and divorced are likely
to obtain a lesser measure of support than that accorded to couples and
that wives give more support to their husbands than the latter give to
their wives (Miles, 1988). The nature and effects of social support are
discussed in Chapter 4.

Several studies of people living alone have demonstrated their vulnerability to isolation and loneliness and the decline in health that
may ensue. Thus, the elderly living alone (Jerome, 1981; Evers, 1985),
the widowed of both younger and older ages and the recently divorced
are at risk (Stroebe and Stroebe, 1983). Indeed, research shows that it is
a common experience in contemporary urban society to lose contact
with friends after bereavement or divorce. Quite often people appear
to withdraw in crisis and it becomes difficult for the widowed and
divorced to maintain friendships (Hart, 1976; Evason, 1980).

It has been argued that marriage imposes a comparatively greater
strain on the distaff side of the alliance and that consequently wives are
the more vulnerable to stress-rated disorders (Gove, 1979). Contemporary marriage is an unequal relationship and, typically, the husband is
the dominant partner. British studies reveal husbands as exercizing
financial control and making most of the important decisions, while
wives have to do much more of the adjusting (Edgell, 1980). These
facets of a relatively weak situation are conducive to stress in the
housewife (it will be remembered that wives with outside employment
enjoy better health than those who do not). Marital relationships and
the stresses experienced by married women vary according to class,
just as the health of the economically secure widow or divorced
woman is likely to differ favourably from that experienced by women
living alone in poverty. This patterning can be seen in the case of an
important category of women, the mothers who live with their children
but without adult male partners.

Single or lone mothers
No satisfactory term has been devised for the very many mothers who
live alone with their children. The phrase 'single mother' can apply to
the unwedded as well as to the widowed or divorced while 'lone
mother', favoured by some, has connotations of loneliness and desire
for company that may not always apply. But whatever collective noun
is preferred, the evidence by Blaxter is that 'single' mothers have a
poorer health record than that of mothers living with their spouses.
Blaxter's results are borne out by a number of other studies which have
demonstrated the greater health problems of mothers living without
partners: Burnell and Wadsworth (1981) found that such mothers evaluated their own health on a lower level than did comparable married

women. Stress-related symptoms, such as headaches, anxiety and depression are, especially, more often reported by these mothers than by married ones, and symptoms of other disorders, for example rheumatic conditions, are also more frequently reported by them. Lone mothers consult their doctors more often than do married mothers and take more medicines (Banks *et al.*, 1975; Evason, 1980).

Stress is inherent in the situation of the woman trying to bring up her children alone. A husband may do little but that little helps, and it is a comfort to have someone with whom to discuss the problems that may arise concerning the health, school performance, etc., of the offspring. Moreover, fathers are something more than just another adult on the premises; the majority of them will be concerned about their children's welfare and take a real interest in their upbringing. Mothers living with their children's father do not usually feel so alone as do single mothers, who may feel that no one else has a real interest in their children and that all decisions have to be made alone. The burden of self-recrimination about seemingly wrong decisions also has to be borne alone. In addition, many divorced and never-married mothers experience guilt feelings, however unjustified, for not managing the situation in such a way as to produce a 'real' father for their children. Indeed, the anticipation of such feelings prevents some women from contemplating divorce (Miles, 1988).

Financial hardship and other material disadvantages hit single mothers and their children disproportionately and class has an important bearing here. Women with high educational attainments and qualifications are likely to pursue careers and earn salaries which adequately support them and their children, but these women are in a minority. The majority of divorced and separated women are those who married young and soon had children without obtaining educational or vocational skills and qualifications. These mothers, as well as a large proportion of the never-married ones, are amongst the most disadvantaged. In Britain, about half of the single mothers and their children rely on state benefits for their income, compared to only 5 per cent of two-parent families (Popay *et al.*, 1983). Such women and their children are less likely than others to live in owner-occupied housing but more likely frequently to move home because they lack security of tenure (Allan, 1985).

Insecurity, financial pressures, lack of adult company in the home and the burden of bringing up children alone, all constitute stressful conditions which take their toll on the health of women who find themselves in the situation of being 'single parents'.

Cigarette smoking and alcohol consumption

Cigarette smoking

It was pointed out at the beginning of this chapter that cause of death is a somewhat problematic notion. 'Lung cancer', or 'bronchial carcinoma' may be entered on a death certificate, but the illness may have been due to cigarette smoking which might in turn have been prompted by stresses and pressure in the social and psychological circumstances of the deceased person's life.

Smoking is widely regarded as one of the most important contributors to ill health in the population. It has been demonstrated to be a major cause of death from cancers of the lung, lip and larynx (90 per cent of deaths due to these diseases are attributed to smoking), as well as from heart disease, bronchitis and obstructive lung disease (Merrison, 1979; Doyal *et al.*, 1983; Balarajan *et al.*, 1985). Moreover, cigarette smoking increases the risk of a wide range of other diseases, including cancers of the cervix, bladder and pancreas, and it has been calculated that heavy smokers have a 76 per cent higher risk of developing chronic illness, than non-smokers (Balarajan *et al.*, 1985). Not surprisingly, increasing attention has been paid, especially over the last three decades, to smoking habits and many educational campaigns have been conducted in the United States, Britain and elsewhere in Western Europe, aimed at persuading people to stop, or never to start, smoking (Department of Health and Social Security, 1976; U.S. Department of Health, Education and Welfare, 1979).

The main sources of information on people's smoking habits are surveys based on self-reports (additional information derives from the sales figures of the tobacco industry). The problems associated with relying on self-reports were noted previously, but additional difficulties arise with surveys on smoking, individuals usually being very aware that society at large, and health professionals in particular, disapprove of this habit. People in the 1980s who answer survey questions have been exposed to much publicity about the harmful effects of cigarette smoking, and know that the habit is widely considered to be 'anti-social' damaging not only to the smokers' health, but that of non-smokers exposed to a smoke-laden atmosphere. In such circumstances, respondents may well under-report their smoking habits. The British *Health and Life-style Survey* (Cox *et al.*, 1987) asked detailed questions about individual smoking habits. Table 1.11 shows the percentages of women and men in Britain who are regular smokers. The figures for men include cigar and pipe smoking (35% of men of all ages, taken collectively, smoke cigarettes only). According to these statistics, a higher proportion of men than of women, in each age bracket, smoke

Table 1.11 Current regular smokers (percentages)

Age	Women	Men
18–29	35	38
30–39	34	41
40–49	34	46
50–59	37	42
60–69	28	40
70–79	16	35
80+	8	26
All ages	31	41

Source: Golding, 1987.

regularly, the gender difference being smallest in the youngest age group. Cigarette consumption was also found to be higher among men that among women, the latter smoking fewer cigarettes a day and being more likely to use the filter variety (Golding, 1987). Similar patterns have been reported in the United States (U.S. Department of Health, Education and Welfare, 1979).

During the last twenty years, a sustained reduction in smoking among people of both sexes, has been noted in Britain and the United States, although the reduction in the case of women was considerably less than for men (Waldron, 1982a). For example, in Britain between 1972 and 1984, the proportion of women who smoked cigarettes declined by 22 per cent: the rate for men fell by approximately half as much again (Office of Health Economics, 1987).

Thus the difference between the proportion of female and male smokers has narrowed. Waldron (1983a) has rightly argued that, traditionally, smoking was more common among men than among women in many parts of the world, a factor which undoubtedly contributed to the higher mortality rates of men, but that today the pattern of smoking is dramatically altered. For example, in Britain between 1972 and 1984, the number of female smokers expressed as a proportion of the equivalent males has risen from 86 to 96 per cent; indeed, the sex difference appears to be reversing in the younger (16–18) age groups among whom a higher proportion of girls (32%) than of boys (29%) are smokers (Office of Health Economics, 1987).

The smoking habits of schoolchildren are of particular interest if only because habits acquired early may be the more difficult to shake off in later years.

Table 1.12 shows the smoking behaviour of schoolchildren in England and Wales in 1984; subsequently published figures show a reduc-

Table 1.12 Smoking behaviour among school children in England and Wales by sex and school year, 1984 (percentages)

Smoking status	Boys						Girls					
	1st	2nd	3rd	4th	5th	All	1st	2nd	3rd	4th	5th	All
Have never smoked	75	52	41	32	23	44	76	55	48	30	25	46
Tried smoking once	17	28	25	28	22	24	16	26	22	23	21	22
Used to smoke	4	10	9	14	14	11	3	9	9	13	14	10
Smoke occasionally	4	7	12	10	10	9	4	8	12	9	11	9
Smoke regularly	0	3	12	17	31	13	1	2	9	24	28	13

Source: Dobbs and Marsh, 1984.

tion by 1985 of 7 per cent for boys, but hardly any (less than 1 per cent) for girls (Goddard and Ikin, 1986).

What prompts young girls to start smoking? Influences on the smoking behaviour of schoolchildren were studied by Anne Charlton and Valerie Blair (1989) who found that parental smoking was the factor most significantly related to the uptake of smoking in girls; interestingly, this was less so for boys. It is possible that girls spend more of their time within the home and, tending to be conformists, are the more likely to be influenced by their parents. For boys, the most important factor was peer smoking, also a major influence on girls, although less so than parental example. Peer pressure has long been regarded as an important element in the decision to smoke, and Charlton and Blair noted that 'a best friend who smoked' was an important influence on girls who, in addition, popularly believed that cigarettes could calm their nerves and aid them in keeping their weight down. These latter considerations would not loom so large in the thinking of boys, but more research is needed to explain why the recent reduction in smoking by schoolchildren is so much more marked among boys than girls.

Turning to the adult population, the questions of why women smoke, and why the fall in their smoking rates is much less than that of men, admit of no easy answers. It is possible that as more women work, and their career opportunities broaden, women are exposed to pressures previously experienced mainly by men. For example, the Office of Health Economics argues (OHE, 1987, p. 54):

it might be predicted that improvements in women's career opportunities could be associated with an increase in the prevalence of those types of morbidity in which competitiveness, time urgency and other facets of Type A behaviour play a causal role.

Table 1.13 Prevalence of cigarette smoking in Great Britain in 1984 according to job. Percentage smoking, aged 16 and over

Job status	Women	Men
Professional	15	17
Employers and managers	29	29
Intermediate and junior non-manual	28	30
Skilled manual and own-account non professional	37	40
Semi-skilled manual and personal service	37	45
Unskilled manual	36	49
All	32	36

Source: OPCS, 1986.

This explanation, however, does not account for the high proportion of smokers among unskilled female workers to whom the exigencies of 'competitiveness' and 'time urgency' would scarcely apply.

Table 1.13 shows the class-related nature of smoking and points especially to the markedly lower rates of smoking among professional people, male and female, *vis-à-vis* workers in all other groups. In fact, smoking can be said to rise in inverse proportion to social position; the lower the status, the higher the rate of smoking. Trends over the decade prior to 1984 show that the proportion of smokers declined in most groups, but the decline was most marked in the professional group.

Smoking also varies according to marital status; for example, in Britain, recently, 49 per cent of widowed, divorced and separated women smoked, but the respective figures were 37 per cent for married women and 34 per cent for the never-married (OPCS, 1986).

If smoking is shown to be related to social class and marital status, it may well be that the key to women's smoking is to be found therein.

Women in the lower socio-economic groupings experience more hardship and more stress than are met with by those in better circumstances, factors which may well account for the greater prevalence of smoking among these groupings. Similarly, widows and divorced women are likely to find themselves in a more stressful situation than are either married or single women and consequently may smoke the more. Bryan Turner, however, postulates (Turner, 1987, p. 108) that as the:

> social status of women begins to approximate that of men in terms of their citizenship rights (especially in employment, education and welfare) then we may expect the disease categories of men and women to become increasingly parallel.

According to this view, women take up habits, previously formed mainly by men, exactly as their life-styles and the pressures on them become more similar to those of men. To some women, cigarette smoking may have appeared as one of the good things that men enjoy and which they, too, wished to experience. This would indicate a 'time lag' between female and male smoking behaviour, and that as men reduce smoking, so eventually will women. Sargent (1979) argued that because women are the less powerful, subordinated group in society, there is a tendency for them to emulate the behaviour of the dominant male group; thus women started to smoke following widespread male smoking, and, possibly, will reduce the habit, following male patterns.

It is also noteworthy that women share with schoolgirls the belief that smoking is 'calming'; stressful situations, which women experience in abundance, call for calming measures. The connection between smoking and the desire to reduce weight is little understood, but there is considerable pressure on women to be slim (see Chapter 4). Jockeys, for whom weight control is crucial, smoke cigars to dull the appetite.

Some writers focus attention on the social acceptability of female smoking; for example, American researcher Ingrid Waldron argues (Waldron, 1983b, p. 1113) that:

> sex differences in cigarette smoking have decreased during the recent period in Western countries at the same time as the dangers of cigarette smoking have become more evident and more widely publicized. It appears that the major determinant of sex differences in cigarette smoking has been the changing patterns of social acceptability of cigarette smoking for men and women and these patterns appear to have varied independently of knowledge of the health risks involved.

Certainly, there does not seem to be the marked gender difference in acceptability of smokers that exists, for example, in respect of drinking problems: male smokers are nó more acceptable than female smokers today.

The increase in female smoking and the decrease of sex differences in smoking, are reflected in the pattern of lung cancer. The sex ratio for death from lung cancer showed a peak around 1960 when male death rates were nine times greater than female death rates in England & Wales, but by 1979 the male death rate had fallen to four times the female death rate (Lopez, 1984). This was due to the rise in female lung cancer mortality. Figures on new cases of lung cancer show that the disease is rising alarmingly in women (in 1983 in England & Wales, there was a 36 per cent increase over the total for 1975), while steadily declining in men (OHE, 1987).

Alcohol consumption

Surveying the literature on alcohol consumption, it is striking to find that comparatively little research was conducted on female drinkers before 1970. While research on patterns of male drinking and alcohol dependence was very large, Birchmore and Walderman (1979) report that they could find only 28 English-language studies on women alcoholics, published between 1929 and 1970. Likewise, studies of the impact of alcohol on the body and studies of treatment methods have been predominantly concerned with men. This preoccupation of researchers with male drinkers was a reflection of substantially higher levels of known alcohol consumption by men compared to that by women (OHE, 1987). Traditionally, regular consumption of alcohol was socially acceptable for men but not for women, and hard drinking and dependence on alcohol were seen as mainly male patterns of behaviour. The extent of female drinking that occurred, especially as much of it may have been hidden and unreported, is now difficult to assess.

During the 1970s, much media attention was paid to women's drinking. According to Robinson (Robinson, 1979, p. 110):

> There is hardly any wide circulation newspaper, magazine or professional health journal which has not carried an article on the 'problem' of women and alcohol. It is not a matter of more women suddenly becoming alcoholic, but of an increased awareness of, and willingness to take seriously, the alcohol-related problems of women.

As interest awakened, alcohol consumption of women became more seriously researched.

Studies show that social attitudes have changed very slowly: while the drinking of alcohol by women has become more socially acceptable, drunkenness in women has not, though society maintains a degree of tolerance towards male intoxication. Normative standards have changed little in this respect; for example, Dight (1976), surveying Scottish drinking habits, found that both drinking and drunkenness were tolerated less in women than in men. According to her study, the vast majority of Scottish people (93 per cent of women and 90 per cent of men) thought that a drunken woman was a 'far more disgusting sight' than a drunken man. Similar findings of less tolerant attitudes towards drinking problems in women were noted by other researchers, for example, by Corrigan (1980) and Knupfer (1982) in Canada, and by Cartwright et al. (1975) in South London. One implication of the very negative attitudes towards women's intoxication may well be a considerable under-reporting of alcohol consumption by women respon-

Table 1.14 Categories of drinker by age and sex, in Britain (percentages)

Drinking status	Males			Females		
	18–39	*40–59*	*60+*	*18–39*	*40–59*	*60+*
Always non-drinker or						
only very occasional	8	13	22	23	32	54
Ex-drinker	5	8	10	6	5	5
Regular drinker:						
None 'last-week'	9	11	9	17	11	9
Light	27	23	35	27	28	19
Moderate	44	40	22	27	24	14
Heavy	8	5	3	1	–	–

Source: Blaxter, 1987b, p. 111.

dents in surveys – not only by women who think they drink 'too much', but by all women. It is, in any case, difficult to collect accurate information about drinking habits, and it is necessary to rely on a variety of sources. In the course of the British *Health and Life-style Survey*, information on alcohol consumption was collected by asking people whether they drank at all, and if so, regularly, or on special occasions only, and by asking them to define their own drinking as light, moderate or heavy. In addition, enquiries were made about past drinking and about alcohol consumption during the seven days prior to the interviews (Blaxter, 1987b). The findings (Table 1.14) show that a considerably higher proportion of women than men were non-drinkers or light drinkers, and that only very few women admitted to consuming alcohol in the quantity defined as amounting to 'heavy' drinking.

In this survey, as elsewhere in recent studies, definitions of 'heavy', 'light' or 'moderate' drinking apply different standards to women and men on the grounds that there are gender differences in the physiological effects of alcohol consumption. Evidence suggests that a given amount of alcohol carries higher risk of physical harm for women and that prolonged heavy drinking is more damaging for women than for men. Women's body size is smaller and the female body contains less water than the male body, thus alcohol becomes more diluted in the male system (Shaw, 1980).

Alcohol consumption is age-related; women over 60 are more likely to be abstainers than younger women; women under 40 are more likely to be regular drinkers.

Trends over time are difficult to establish. The General Household Survey in Britain monitored drinking habits since 1978, and its findings indicate a small increase in the proportion of women who are regular drinkers. There are also indications that alcohol-related problems are increasing in women: growing numbers of women are admitted to hospitals with drinking problems, the number of alcohol-related criminal offences has increased (drinking and driving, drunkenness in public places), more women attend alcoholism counselling services, and the proportion of female members of AA (Alcoholics Anonymous) has increased, especially in the United States and Canada (Shaw, 1980). As Robinson suggested, some of these statistics may be influenced by a greater readiness on the part of women with drink problems to come forward, and by changes in police attitudes in dealing with female offenders, so that any real increase in women's drinking is less than appears. That as may be, but surveys indicate no reduction in alcohol consumption, and according to the Office of Health Economics (OHE, 1987),

> the main cause for concern to emerge from the data is the relatively high and unchanging prevalence of heavy alcohol consumption among young women aged 18–24 years.

Who are the heavy drinkers? Why do they drink? What are their problems? The information is patchy. Part of the difficulty in obtaining an overall picture of women and alcohol is that definitions of heavy drinkers vary. Some experts would argue that any regular drinking is potentially harmful, while others regard light drinking as harmless, even, possibly, beneficial. Women drinkers themselves also vary a great deal in what they view as problem drinking. Nevertheless, some suggestive findings have emerged. According to *The Health and Lifestyle Survey* (Blaxter 1987b), women with employment outside of their homes are more likely to be 'moderate' or 'heavy' drinkers than are housewives without such paid employment. Moreover, drinking would seem to be related to occupation with women in professional, managerial, and other non-manual employment being more likely to be regular drinkers than those working in manual jobs. Other studies likewise indicate that people working in certain occupations are especially exposed to drinking. An obvious example is provided by the employees of public houses and clubs for whom drink is readily available and the nature of the job such that to refuse a drink can seem churlish. A large number of women work in British 'pubs': indeed, in 1978, these establishments employed twice as many women as men (Shaw, 1980). Journalism and other media positions, advertizing, representative work, managerial and executive positions and professions such as medicine, have all been associated with drinking habits higher than average, and the proportion of women in these occupations has increased. A detailed analysis of three national surveys over a fifteen-year period (Filmore, 1984) shows that employed women, especially in the 21–29 age groups, are the ones most likely to become heavy drinkers and that the proportion of such drinkers is increasing in North America and Britain.

However, the alcohol consumption and alcohol-related problems of housewives should not be minimized. Studies of women receiving treatment for alcohol dependence reveal that there are many housewives among them and that their drinking patterns are different from those of women in paid employment. Eileen Corrigan found that many of the women receiving treatment did much of their drinking alone, while others drink their usual quantity only when with close friends and even change friends to accommodate their drinking (Corrigan, 1987, pp. 162–163). She noted that more than a third of a sample of alcoholic women coming to treatment said that they were attempting to hide their drinking. Others, also, have noted that women who become dependent on alcohol often report a pattern of solitary drinking in the home (Saunders, 1980). This pattern may be due to social disapproval of drunkenness in women, fear of exposure and stigma encouraging secrecy.

Unlike the employed women who drink in company and become regular drinkers at an early age, those who drink alone at home, become dependent and attempt to hide it, are likely to be somewhat older women. Alcoholic women tend to enter into treatment at the age of 40–45 and report the beginning of symptoms as occurring shortly before.

A number of factors may play a part in home drinking by females and consequent alcohol dependence. The purchase of alcohol has become easier and more convenient, with supermarkets obtaining licences to sell alcohol. It is socially more acceptable for women to buy alcohol along with the groceries in supermarkets, than to go to special shops selling drinks only. Advertisements increasingly aim at women drinkers and may, as intended, have an impact on women's purchasing, and drinking, alcohol. Advertizing in women's magazines for 'female drinks', i.e. table wines, sherry, liqueurs and vermouths, has gained prominence and large amounts of advertizing expenditure are directed to attracting women to alcohol (National Council of Women, 1976).

There are, probably, many diverse social and psychological reasons for some women becoming dependent on alcohol. Researchers suggest that the lack of companionship and support that many housewives experience, and feelings of non-achievement and frustration may lead women to drink (Shaw, 1980). Attempts to escape from conflicts that have no solutions may be a factor (Gomberg, 1976). It is also of interest that there is a significant correlation between divorce or separation and alcohol dependence, a considerably higher proportion of alcoholic women being divorced or separated than the corresponding proportion of the female population generally. Married and widowed women have a lower proportion of alcoholics among them. It has been suggested that difficult marital relationships and a tendency towards finding escape in drink, may interact and aggravate each other in a vicious circle which is finally broken by divorce at a time when dependence on alcohol has set in (Shaw, 1980). It is also possible that loss of a husband through separation or divorce greatly reduces women's self-esteem, and that for some women coping with loss and humiliation is helped by drinking.

Regular alcohol consumption among young, employed women may well be due to quite different pressures, connected with work, and efforts to behave as men do, in a man's world.

2

Concepts of health and illness

Concepts of health

Health means different things to different people. On being questioned, many are unable clearly to define health and illness although they can say readily enough whether they regard themselves as healthy or not. Such is the common finding of social researchers. People have little difficulty in defining their overall health as good or not so good, nor in distinguishing between the states of being healthy, and being ill: it is part of the human experience for people to consider and try to make sense of the events, misfortunes and ailments which affect them. To feel healthy or sick is a personal experience but concepts of health and illness are learnt by drawing on the accumulated knowledge of the relevant culture. Sociologists argue that in every society there are accepted standards of 'normal' health and fitness which govern its members' thinking about their condition. How these norms develop, how they are learnt and applied and what are regarded as deviations therefrom are matters of great interest to social observers (Freidson, 1975a; Miles, 1978).

Lay concepts of health have excited much research interest. A pioneering study was that conducted by Claudine Herzlich (1973) in France where she interviewed 80 middle-class men and women. She demonstrated that their health concepts could be divided into three groups: the first, saw health as what she termed health-in-a-vacuum, i.e. an absence of illness 'something quite independent of the person, something impersonal' (p. 56); the second, thought of it more in terms of a good constitution, a 'reserve of health' innate or cultivated which endures despite episodes of illness; for the third group, health was a condition of equilibrium, a notion which Herzlich herself regards as poorly defined but which can be applied to the 'normal' condition of a healthy, well-functioning individual feeling at ease both bodily and emotionally. It would have been useful had the research differentiated between the male and female responses but that was not one of its purposes.

Some subsequent researchers sought to ascertain whether people view health positively, the possession of a healthy mind in a healthy body, or negatively, as the absence of illness, the condition of there being 'nothing wrong'.

In fact, past research on lay concepts was concerned with a number of issues, studied from a variety of perspectives, so that the task of summarizing and assessing the relevant findings has proved far from straightforward. Many investigators started from the assumption that modern, Western, scientific medicine, now increasingly called 'biomedicine', constitutes the only right and valid knowledge and endeavoured to ascertain how much of that knowledge was assimilated by lay people and what traditional or other beliefs of theirs hindered that process. A frequent objective of such studies was to help medical practitioners in their attempt to convince people that medical advice was best and that prescribed treatment should be followed. It is only comparatively recently that researchers have begun to explore lay concepts of health and illness as valuable source material for the understanding of individual and social experiences. For example, Stacey (Stacey, 1988, p. 142) takes people's ideas

> as logical and valid in their own right, although they may not be consonant with biomedical science or with any other organised healing system. Ordinary people, in other words, develop explanatory theories to account for their material, social and bodily circumstances. These they apply to themselves as individuals, but in developing them they draw on all sorts of knowledge and wisdom, some of it derived from their own experience, some of it handed on by word of mouth, other parts of it derived from highly trained practitioners.

If the problem of assessing past research on lay concepts resides in the multiplicity of its aims and assumptions the difficulty does not end there. Some researchers failed to make clear the gender, class or other attributes of their samples; others studied only men, or women, of one or another particular social background, rendering generalizations and comparisons far from easy. Indeed, the richest data on lay beliefs are frequently to be found in very detailed studies conducted with small samples and necessarily limited in scope. Many of the investigators who restricted themselves to female respondents had regard to the greater accessibility of women, many of whom are at home during the day. In any case, research with subjects of both sexes indicates that women are the more likely to talk freely about health matters (a point which will be discussed subsequently).

A favoured way of studying the health concepts of individuals is by detailed, lengthy and free interviews with small samples. However, one large-scale survey of health and life style in England, Scotland and Wales (Cox *et al.*, 1987) included an investigation of people's health concepts and their attitudes to health and illness. Some 9000 people were interviewed in their homes and extensively questioned on a variety of health matters including their concepts of health and illness. Describing health in someone else, women (especially those in age groups 18–39 and 40–59) were more likely than men to view it negatively, 'never ill, no disease, never see a doctor' being the category of response most often encountered. Conversely, men (again predominantly in the younger age groups) saw health positively in terms of 'fit, strong, energetic and physically active'. A third category of response, 'able to do a lot, work, socially active' was employed more or less equally by respondents of either sex but here, mostly, by those aged 60+. It could be that these 'virtues' are more ingrained in older people and incorporated by them into images of health and well-being.

Some of the female responses were positive just as those of some of the men were negative. Both sexes tended to describe health in another person in terms either of fitness or the absence of disease, with the women inclining to the latter, more negative, view. However, when asked to describe what it is to be healthy oneself, a different picture emerged.

The predominant concept of health in oneself was a psychological one. To 'feel good, happy, able to cope' was the favoured description employed by both men and women of every age group. According to the author of this part of the survey (Blaxter, 1987d, p. 141)

it is not perhaps surprising that a subjective experience should be described this way, but it is notable that, for themselves, the respondents here were less likely to emphasise either physical fitness or lack of disease, but rather to say that health is defined as being unstressed and unworried, able to cope with life, in tune with the world, and happy.

In another question, respondents were invited to think of (and name) someone who is very healthy. Table 2.1 shows the interesting result that a majority of both sexes, the men especially, nominated a male person in answer to this question. Apparently, rude health is

Table 2.1 Sex of person thought of when asked 'think of someone who is very healthy' (percentages)

Sex of respondent	Sex of person thought of		
	Male	Female	'Can't think of anyone'
Male	66	17	17
Female	47	35	18

Source: Cox *et al.*, 1987.

much more a male characteristic in the eyes of most men and of a large proportion of women too.

Notions of health and the meanings attached to health by individuals are much influenced by their social standing and material circumstances. Social and economic position are major determinants of health and the volume of ill health experienced by individuals, in turn, influences the ways in which they think about health and illness. Moreover, the nature of the work people do and the degree of control that they are able to exercise over their jobs, their daily lives and their relationships are also reflected in their perceptions of health and illness. This was demonstrated by Jocelyn Cornwell (1984) in her study of working-class people in Bethnal Green, an inner-city suburb of London. Her respondents saw themselves as having little control over their work and of other aspects of their daily lives and this acquiescent attitude was paralleled in their views of health and illness as likewise being matters beyond their control.

A number of other studies offer confirmatory evidence of the relationship between social class and health concepts. Blaxter and Patterson (1982) found that women from working-class, socially disadvantaged, backgrounds in Scotland tended to define health in a negative and largely functional way as the absence of illness and the ability to carry on. It is hardly surprising that the experience of ill health and its attendant disruption of daily functioning, in somewhat harsh material circumstances, induces in those who have undergone it a negatory view of health as the condition of being able to perform one's customary duties.

Despite the evidence so far adduced, it is nevertheless the case that the interplay between social class, gender and health beliefs is complex. This was demonstrated by Calnan's study carried out in London, in the course of which women from both working-class and professional backgrounds were interviewed (Calnan and Johnson, 1985; Calnan, 1987). When concepts of health were linked to individuals' own health, no major social class differences appeared; however, when women talked about health in the abstract, there was evidence of class differences (Calnan, 1987, p. 33):

> being 'fit', 'strong', 'active' and 'taking exercise' were commonly referred to by middle-class women as elements of being healthy, but these were rarely mentioned by working-class women. On the other hand, working-class women tended to emphasise the importance of 'never being ill' and the functional requirements of living, such as 'getting through the day'.

Thus, for example, one working-class woman said (p. 33):

> I mean, when you can't do nothing – just lying in bed. Yes, it's when I can't do nothing, when I can't eat – yeah – be them sort of things that would make me think I was really ill. I mean, I've had a cold but I can still get up and do my work and I can see to the children, but if it's I can't get out of bed – then I am ill.

More research is required before all the complexities of the correlation between class, gender and health concepts can be better understood. In particular, more comparative data on the differences between male and female concepts would be of value, since this aspect has tended to be neglected by some researchers in the field.

If anything, even less attention has been paid to the health beliefs of minority ethnic groups living in contemporary Western societies yet information on the culture of such groups, besides its intrinsic worth, would increase understanding among the indigenous majority from whom such groups may differ.

In an interesting study, Caroline Currer (1986) discussed the health concepts of Pathan women from the North-West frontier of Pakistan who had migrated to England. Pathan women are zealous Muslims and strong adherents to the practice of purdah, the system by which women are secluded from men and from public life. Currer (Currer, 1986, p. 189) found that

> Pathan women viewed both health and illness, happiness and unhappiness as part of the natural order, as a part and risk of living. Any feelings that to be healthy was an overall aim or ideal in life was lacking (although health was valued when it occurred).

Notions of health and illness for Pathan women were strongly linked to their ability to work (p. 189):

> the women's value, in their own eyes and those of their community, lay in their ability to care for their husbands and children and manage the home

and they considered themselves healthy while they could carry out such tasks.

Concepts of illness

Whatever meaning is given to health by lay people, ill health represents a breakdown in the normal, expected state of health and well-being, a situation when things go wrong, a deviation from how things should be, and usually are (Miles, 1978). Lay people think about illness in a variety of ways; Herzlich (1973) found that her French respondents held three kinds of conceptions of illness, all developed by individuals in a social context. She termed these conceptions as follows: firstly, 'illness as destructive' meaning that for some people, illness represented inactivity, exclusion from social roles and the giving up of interests (as one respondent said: 'you feel almost left out of society'; p. 105; secondly, 'illness as liberator in the sense that it represents a lessening of burdens and a rest from problems and responsibilities'; and thirdly, 'illness as an "occupation", which people prepare for and learn and actively pursue'.

Not only the meaning of illness, but the form it takes is classified by lay people, who need, as do professional practitioners, classificatory categories in order to explain it. Classification can be developed in different ways by different social groups. For example, working-class people in the London Borough of Bethnal Green followed a tripartite classification, according to Cornwell's study (1984, pp. 130–131 and 151): 'normal illness' was what most people were expected to get sometime, such as infectious diseases in childhood, or colds and flu in winter; 'real illness' meant major disabling and life-threatening diseases; and 'health problems which are not illness' were those associated with natural processes, such as ageing or the reproductive cycle, and also mental health problems such as depression and anxiety.

The category of health problems, which cause pain, distress, and much suffering, but are not perceived as genuine illness, is especially important for women because it includes problems inherent in menstruation, childbirth, pregnancy and menopause and also because women suffer far more than men do from such conditions as depression, anxiety and agoraphobia.

It is interesting to observe that when talking about illness Cornwell's respondents meant physical illness: indeed, she quotes one of them as saying:

> depression ... is not an illness it is a health problem and the person who has it has to help themselves out of it.

Others, too, saw anxiety and depression as states of mind, consigned
to the category of 'health problems that are not illnesses'.

It might be argued that the stigma traditionally attaching to mental
illness (and persistent even today) and the former practice of segregat-
ing the mentally ill from the community created a climate in which the
subject became unmentionable and that this social taboo still surrounds
it. It has been a consistent finding of researchers (confirmed by the
experiences of health practitioners) that lay people have uncertain,
often ambivalent and contradictory, views about the meaning of mental disturbance, and whether to regard it as illness or not. In a recent
study of women treated for neurotic disorders, it was found that the
women themselves, as well as their relatives, friends and colleagues,
shared the assumption that a 'genuinely' sick person is physically
unwell and that it is very questionable whether depression or agoraphobia should be regarded as illness (Miles, 1988).

Educational and class background are likely to influence thinking on
these issues: middle-class people of higher educational attainments are
more likely than working-class people to regard mental illness as 'real'.
It was from middle-class women that Calnan heard references made to
being depressed or unhappy when talking about illness. In fact, one
woman is quoted as describing illness in just these terms saying,
'depression itself is an illness isn't it?' (Calnan, 1987, p. 34).

Studies from the United States also show that occupation, and the
'social circle' a person moves in, tend greatly to influence whether
mental disturbance is seen as an illness or not. According to a study of
patients of New York psychotherapy clinics, members of some social
circles had more 'psychiatric sophistication' than others and were more
likely to define mental disturbance as 'real' illness, similar to physical
illnesses (Kadushin, 1968). Such 'sophistication' was closely related not
only to educational level and social class, but also to type of occupation: for instance, people working in showbusiness, advertizing,
communications and teaching were more likely than engineers,
businessmen or lawyers to view mental distress as illness.

Attributing causes to illness

It has been shown that people categorize illness and make decisions as
to which problems can, and which cannot, be so regarded. Also, it is
important for people to understand and be able to explain to themselves why they have become ill. What caused it? How could it have
been avoided?

When the presence of illness is established, the usual first desire is to put a name to it (Balint, 1964): having named it, or been told what it is, individuals begin the process of assessing what has befallen them. For some, a causal explanation is sought in a cry against fate: 'Why me?' 'What have I done to be singled out for this misfortune?' Others will look for physical causes, remembering a recent contact with someone who kept on sneezing or saying vaguely, 'It must have been something I ate'. Always it is necessary to find answers for if none is forthcoming or none is acceptable, then the events in one's life have no meaning and nothing can be done to stave off future disasters. This is a depressing, indeed a frightening conclusion, and not surprisingly people, as they have throughout history, seek to interpret natural phenomena and struggle to make sense of their experiences. In this they rely on the sum of knowledge and beliefs which exist in the society of their time and place. According to (Herzlich and Pierret, 1986, p. 73)

> In so-called 'traditional' societies, illness, a crucial but incomprehensible event for both the individual and the group, has always given rise to questioning and interpretations which go beyond the body itself. The problems of causality of biological illness are therefore at the heart of any society's system of beliefs and of the data which anthropologists must observe and theorise about.

Little is known from research about gender differences in explanations for illness. It is likely that women, more often than men, think about and seek to explain illness in themselves and their families. Women have higher rates of morbidity and suffer the pain and discomfort attendant upon childbirth and menstrual processes, experiences which serve to focus their interest upon illness and the reasons for it. In her study of working-class women, conducted in Scotland, Mildred Blaxter (Blaxter, 1983, p. 69) found

> many examples of the women worrying over symptoms, consulting again and again, because (although they had been given a diagnosis), they had not been given a cause or at least one which they found acceptable.

The women in her study talked a great deal about causes of diseases and Table 2.2 shows the most frequently mentioned categories of cause. Infection, including infectious diseases of childhood, was the most mentioned cause and one closely associated with the environment. The infection–environmental connection is frequently met with in lay explanations of illness because of the tendency to assume that germs become more widespread and more dangerous in given climatic and material conditions. Blaxter also explained that (Blaxter, 1983, p. 63):

Table 2.2 Categories of cause mentioned by 46 women. The number of instances in each case is given

1 Infection	126
2 Heredity of familial tendencies	55
3 Agents in the environment: 'poisons', working conditions, climate	48
4 Secondary to other diseases	42
5 Stress, strain and worry	27
6 Caused by childbearing, menopause	27
7 Secondary to trauma or to surgery	25
8 Neglect, the constraints of poverty	19
9 Inherent susceptibility, individual and not hereditary	18
10 Behaviour, own responsibility	18
11 Ageing, natural degeneration	14

Source: Blaxter, 1983, p. 62.

the popularity of 'external' causes – 'something in the water', 'dampness in these houses' – appeared to represent a very natural desire on the women's part to allot 'blame'. To find a cause in the environment was more acceptable than to locate responsibility in one's own body, and an obvious way of rationalising the unknown. In any case, the women's lives truly presented many candidates for an environmental explanation of ill health – an unkind climate, often poor housing and work in unpleasant conditions.

Data from other researchers confirm the general preference for explaining physical illness by the attribution of external causes. Thus, the study of Pill and Stott (on mothers of children in South Wales), also found that the women most often mentioned 'germs', 'bugs' and 'viruses' when talking about causes of illness. (Pill and Stott, 1982).

This popular preference for external causes is understandable, not just for the reasons given but because alternative explanations may confront the uncomfortable possibility of an individual's own behaviour having caused or contributed to the illness, e.g. through neglect of hygiene or by smoking and drinking. Stress, strain and worry are other explanations which find favour (see Table 2.2) since these, too, locate the source of the problem outside personal control. The Scottish women spoke of strain at the workplace, the worry of a dying husband, and the shock of bereavement. In general, Blaxter argued, the thinking of these women about illness causation tended to be influenced by past experiences, both personal and handed down through generations, and that they exhibited 'a liking for continuity, a firm long-term family identity' (Blaxter, 1983, p. 64), sentiments which may explain why heredity and familial tendencies figure so prominently on the list of causes.

Current official policy on health education may well be another factor bearing on women's thinking. Often, women have been the main target of health education campaigns which carry the message that people must take greater responsibility for their health by adopting healthier life-styles and habits in order to lessen the risk of illness (Department of Health and Social Security, 1976). To ensure that healthy habits prevail in the household has long been regarded as an essential part of women's role, particularly in matters of cleanliness and the provision of a suitable diet (Graham, 1984). Advertizing makes the same point; almost always it is a woman who is seen cleansing the toilet or pouring the breakfast cereal.

This general emphasis on women's responsibility for the health of the family puts an extra burden on wives and mothers and increases their potential for blame and guilt. Understandably, they are likely unconsciously to develop explanations for illness which put the blame on factors beyond their control.

Talking in general terms about causes of illness is one thing; explaining why illness has hit one is something else and, when the condition is serious, even life threatening, leads to anguished self-questioning: 'How did I get into this situation?' or, simply, 'Why me?' Perhaps most painful is the struggle to find answers in cases of mental disturbance where issues of individual responsibility, blame and guilt tend to be heightened. A study of women and men treated by psychiatrists for neurotic disorders demonstrated the intensity of their efforts to attribute causes to their condition (Miles, 1988). Women delved deeper, considered a broader range of explanations, and were readier than men to discard facile and superficial solutions. The women looked to internal rather than external causes, tending to locate the origin of their neurotic illness in their own past actions, their relationships and their own bodies. In this, their thinking differed from that of women seeking causes of physical illness in themselves or in others who, as we have seen, wanted causes outside their control. They differed also from men in the same study, who almost exclusively found explanations for their neurosis in external factors, namely work and past physical illness (Table 2.3).

The attribution of internal factors to illness carries with it the implication of avoidability, with responsibility and therefore blame resting with the ill person. Many women suffering from depression, anxiety or agoraphobia blame themselves for these problems: in the study referred to above (Miles, 1988, p. 27) one young woman said:

Table 2.3 Most frequently considered causes of neurosis

	Women (n = 65)	Men (n = 20)
Unsatisfactory marriage	32	–
Past actions	25	–
Hormone changes: PMT, menopause, postnatal	25	–
Unsatisfactory family relationships	18	–
Caring for sick, disabled or elderly relative	13	–
Adverse life events	11	4
Childhood experiences	8	1
Problems at work	3	11
Physical illness or surgery	3	10

Source: Miles, 1988.

I was pregnant when I was 16, my boy-friend was 18, his parents made him say he'd have nothing to do with me. My parents wanted me to have an abortion, but I said no, I was going to have the baby. When Nicky was born I was ill, then depressed. I wasn't really ready to have a child then. I ran away for nearly two years and left the baby with my mother, it was terrible for her. I think when I decided to have the baby, and not to have an abortion, I started all my nervous troubles. I love Nicky now and try to make up for it, but still, I caused my own troubles ...

A woman in Cornwell's study (Cornwell, 1984, p. 152) who suffered from bouts of depression, as did her mother, and who might therefore have sought to blame 'heredity' instead thought, like her mother, that the problem lay with failure to act responsibly in situations for which she was to blame. (It seems probable that although the daughter had not inherited the illness she had certainly adopted her mother's attitude to it.) After losing her baby the daughter reported that she:

'...couldn't quite get back to what I consider normal. I couldn't get back to the way I wanted to feel and I should've felt, so I went to the doctor's and he gave me some [tranquillizers].' Both mother and daughter looked inward for the causes of their depression.

Feelings of guilt and the self-examination attendant upon the 'why me?' question are also characteristic of women who have undergone a miscarriage. In fact, miscarriage is a common occurrence in the sense that the majority of human conceptions do not result in the birth of a

live baby. Even so, in more advanced societies today there is a strong
expectation that pregnancy and childbirth will proceed smoothly with
the consequence that miscarriage, like illness, requires an explanation.
According to a study of women who had experienced a miscarriage,
there is a strong tendency among them to locate the cause in themselves and to indulge in self-blame: they cited their errors of behaviour,
their imperfect mental attitudes or the inadequacies of their bodies
(Oakley *et al.*, 1984).

> Was God punishing me for not loving the baby enough? Was it
> His way of showing me just how special each child is? . . . I believe
> it was meant to be. That there was some special reason for it.
> Perhaps my changed attitude to life and children was the only
> reason? [p. 112]

> . . . although my GP said this wasn't the cause, I did for a short
> time blame overwork for the miscarriage. Also, during the latter
> couple of weeks of the pregnancy I was worried (unnecessarily)
> about my husband's business. [p. 115]

> I have to convince myself it was some deformity on the growth of
> the fetus, although I have in the past blamed it on any number of
> things, drinking, dieting before conception, allowing myself to
> get tired, lifting a heavy weight in the first weeks. . . [p. 116]

The authors of this study noted a curious feature of their respondent's
self-blame, found also among people seeking the causes of their mental
disturbance, namely that enjoyable experiences were much more often
considered as possible causes than those which were not enjoyed.
Such experiences included pleasurable work, good holidays, and indulgence in food and drink. This possibly reflects a lingering puritani-
cal ethic that pleasure is sinful and invites retribution.

It is of interest to observe that people trying to find the causes of
their physical or mental problems seldom consider that these causes
might be located in the wider social structure. The various studies
which have explored women's attribution of causes to illness have
failed to note them considering any connection between broad social
issues and ill-health. Thus, women may explain ill-health in themselves by blaming environmental factors such as poor housing, or
harsh domestic duties or the prolonged nursing of sick or disabled
family members, without questioning why such tasks should fall to the
lot of women and without raising the political issues of re-housing or
the provision of better social services for women in their situations.

Health or illness?

Pregnancy

A consideration of popular notions of health and illness reveals that concepts and perceptions are seldom clear-cut and firmly held but, on the contrary, are ill-defined, elastic and often elusive. To be sure, people have firm ideas as to the nature of some sorts of disease (for example that a life-threatening condition is a 'real' illness) but they are vague and vacillatory about many others. Included in this latter are the problems associated with the reproductive system of women, particularly pregnancy, about which views are characterized by ambiguity.

It may be said that in late twentieth century Western societies, central to the experience of pregnancy, is this ambiguity as to its nature: is it a state of health or of illness? Women struggle to find an answer, to attach meanings to their experiences and to ascertain the socially approved and appropriate ways to behave. Ambiguity arises from the conflicting messages which reach women: from doctors and other health professionals, from relatives and friends, and from their own bodies. One message assimilated by girls during the early years of gender socialization is that being pregnant is a natural state for women, not an illness, and that having a baby is part of womanhood and femininity. Many women enter pregnancy for the first time holding this view only to be surprised by the opposite message from health professionals, i.e. that pregnancy is a medical condition to be checked and monitored by doctors. Obstetricians in hospital ante-natal clinics treat pregnant women 'as if ill'; Ann Oakley in a study of women's experience of pregnancy and childbirth noted that an average of 13 visits were made by women to doctors, hospitals and clinics during their pregnancy (Oakley, 1981). This conflict between the notion of a 'natural', healthy biological process and the notion of pregnancy as a medical condition is typified by one of her respondents, thus (Oakley, 1981, p. 46):

> It's this concern with medicine that seems to override everything else – the natural process, I mean. I mean it is something women have always been brought up to; everybody knows that, okay, it's painful, having labour and everything, but it's also rewarding; it's the one pain we've been brought up to expect and not to be scared of. Before going to the hospital, pregnancy was a normal, nice condition. I'm not so sure it isn't an illness now.

Uncertainties about the nature of pregnancy are also aroused by the bodily sensations of pain and discomfort which many pregnant women experience. While some women thrive on pregnancy, others feel

Table 2.4 Some pregnancy symptoms (percentages)

Tiredness	93
Vomiting/nausea	86
Frequent urination	82
Sleep disturbance	70
Indigestion	63
Constipation	52

Source: Oakley, 1981, p. 48.

less well than usual and suffer diminished energy. Ann Oakley found that the majority experienced symptoms of one sort or another (Table 2.4).

Some of these symptoms are more likely to occur during the first 3–4 months, others during the latter stages of pregnancy; but the characteristic experience is of the fluctuating nature of the problems. Interestingly, despite the symptoms, most women describe their general state as healthy. Hilary Homans (1985) interviewed 78 women, half of them White British and half of them British women of Punjabi origin. All of the women experienced at least one sort of discomfort while no fewer than 88 per cent reported a variety of disorders. The range of complaints was similar for both groups although the 'Punjabi' women spoke of weakness and tiredness while the 'Whites' stressed heartburn as their main problem. But, as Table 2.5 shows, 75 per cent of the women described their health in positive terms.

Women see themselves as healthy in spite of a measure of discomfort which they see as natural to pregnancy. This was the finding of Hilary Graham and Ann Oakley in their studies of mothers in York and London for whom bearing children was viewed as a 'natural biological process' like other biological processes that occur in women's lives, a process 'rooted in the bodies of women' (Graham and Oakley 1986, p. 101).

By contrast, doctors regard the entire state of pregnancy, and the disorders attendant upon it, as medical concerns and it is this message that is conveyed by them to women. Oakley notes that a large variety of drugs are used in pregnancy, many on doctors' prescriptions.

Doctors have long provided advice and treatment for pregnancy. In the United States, reviewing 150 years of experts' advice to women, Barbara Ehrenreich and Deidre English (1979) observed that the textbook image of the pregnant woman has been of one 'indisposed' throughout the full nine months. Medical advice in the past required a woman (p. 111)

Table 2.5 Women's description of their state of health during pregnancy

Responses	n	Percentage
Positive responses		
Same as usual	6	8
Good/fine	16	20
All right	26	33
Very good/very well	11	14
Negative responses		
Poor	7	9
Not very well	3	4
Rotten/terrible	3	4
Suicidal	1	1
Bit depressed	2	3
Better now	3	4
Total	78	100

Source: Homans, 1985, p. 142.

to avoid all 'shocking, painful or unbeautiful sights', intellectual stimulation, angry or hurtful thoughts and even her husband's alcohol and tobacco breath.

The authors stress that such advice was given to White middle-class women; Black women and White working-class women did not have the time or money to support a cult of invalidism and were regarded by doctors as 'robust' and 'free from uterine disease' (p. 114). Either way, the message conveyed was that doctors are the arbitrators on pregnancy.

Contemporary health professionals also give advice freely, and it certainly seems that a conflict exists between their notions of pregnancy and those of the women concerned. Graham and Oakley argue (1986, p. 99), that there are 'competing ideologies of reproduction', that 'doctors and mothers have a qualitatively different way of looking at the nature, context and management of reproduction'.

However, it would be a simplification of a complex reality to say that all doctors treat pregnancy as a medical condition (i.e. an 'illness'), while mothers invariably think of it as a healthy one: the perspectives of both groups are more complicated. Although women think of pregnancy as natural, they have been greatly influenced by medical teaching; their notions on the nature and context of pregnancy and of the appropriateness of medical intervention have been conditioned by several generations of expert advice. Perceptions and beliefs regarding pregnancy are part of wider perceptions and beliefs as to the nature of health and the role of doctors. Women who habitually turn to doctors with their complaints (and have been encouraged to do so) will incline to doctors as the appropriate experts on the discomforts of pregnancy. Indeed, while women may resent medical intervention in the 'natural' process of pregnancy, they will none the less take exception to any unwillingness by doctors to help them overcome the concomitant discomfort.

Contemporary doctors also, are divided in their views. Among them, obstetricians are the more likely to view pregnancy as a pathological condition (Graham and Oakley, 1986) and the linking of their speciality to gynaecology serves to reinforce the image of reproduction as being in the realm of medicine. By contrast, many, but by no means all, general practitioners view pregnancy as a natural process and consequently outside their purview. Hilary Homans, reporting this division between British doctors, found some refusing to prescribe drugs for pregnant women, insisting that discomfort is normal, and others prepared to prescribe drugs to alleviate symptoms during pregnancy (Homans, 1985).

Advice obtained from the pregnant woman's social network of friends, relatives and workmates is another source of ambiguity, such advice often being contradictory exactly because of the lack of consensus as to the nature of pregnancy. General uncertainties and contradictory views are illustrated by the following quotations from Ann Oakley's study (Oakley, 1981, p. 47):

> I think you should behave as you normally would. Women work out in the fields till they give birth. That's what I keep saying to myself. They give you all these things to do, and it seems ridiculous when most women – probably 95 per cent of women – who have children don't bother.

> I think of it as something abnormal. I can't take it completely in my stride. I'm aware every minute of the day that there's something different about me.

> Well, my sister treats it as normal. She says it's not an illness. She says it's a natural thing. She was hanging up wallpaper, or doing something decorating her beautiful home I think it was, a night or two before her babies were born. She's very much like my mother – she's very healthy and she just has her kids, no trouble, you know. I'm different altogether. I think you should rest and look after yourself. Maybe I'm wrong, I don't know.

Hilary Homans found that white British women differed according to social class in how they dealt with pregnancy and its discomforts. Middle-class women were more inclined than working-class women to turn to their doctors as a first resort with their complaints, although middle-class women were also more questioning and doubtful about drugs, being more aware of possibly harmful side effects. Interestingly, it seems that immigrant groups experience a great deal of pressure to conform to the ways of the host population. Health professionals, together with educational programmes and leaflets, encourage ethnic minority groups to consult doctors and thus their women lean to the medical image of pregnancy at a time when white middle-class women increasingly question it (Homans, 1985).

Menstruation

Menstruation, like pregnancy, is surrounded by ambiguities and uncertainties. Although menstruation is a normal, healthy function of the female body, it causes pain and discomfort; indeed, many women are incapacitated for a few days each month by this natural function. An experience which at the same time is both 'healthy' and painful is confusing and deeply rooted social attitudes enhance the ambiguities.

The medical profession has been as ready to give advice to women on how to deal with menstruation as they have been about pregnancy. In their book on 150 years of experts' advice to women, Ehrenreich and English (1979) quoted several physicians from the early part of the twentieth-century who regarded menstruation as a threat throughout life: 'The doctors assumed that every woman was prepared to set aside a week or five days every month as a period of invalidism.' Dr W. C. Taylor, in his book *A Physician's Counsel to Women in Health and Disease*, gave a warning typical of those found in popular health books of the time:

> We cannot too emphatically urge the importance of regarding these monthly returns as periods of ill-health, as days when the ordinary occupations are to be suspended or modified ... long walks, dancing, shopping, riding and parties should be avoided at this time of month invariably and under all circumstances ...

As late as 1916, Dr Winfield Scott Hall was advising (Ehrenreich and English, 1979, p. 111):

> All heavy exercise should be omitted during the menstrual week ... a girl should not only retire earlier at this time, but ought to stay out of school from one to three days as the case may be, resting the mind and taking extra hours of rest and sleep!

Such advice was addressed primarily to middle-class women while, as the list of activities to be avoided shows, those of the working class were expected to carry on with their duties regardless of painful periods. These early medical opinions seem remote in late twentieth-century Western societies where advertisements for tampons and sanitary towels portray women full of health, undertaking strenuous exercise with a smile, during menstruation.

However Emily Martin argued recently that in contemporary American college texts, menstruation appears as pathological rather than natural and healthy. Terms such as 'degenerate', 'deterioration', 'repair', 'decline' and 'weakened', taken by Martin from current physiological textbooks, place menstruation in the realm of illness. Illustrations in these manuals capture the image of catastrophic disintegration, often being accompanied by yet further words of foreboding like 'ceasing', 'dying', 'expelling' and 'denuding', terms which convery failure and dissolution (Martin, 1989, pp. 47–48). If this image of menstruation impresses itself upon doctors they may, in a number of subtle ways, convey it to their patients. Not surprisingly, many women find it difficult to decide how much discomfort and pain should be regarded as part of normal health and at what point the threshold of illness or the abnormal is crossed.

Women's groups, conducting health courses in the United States and in Britain tend to emphasize that menstruation is a natural, healthy process, and therefore that women should see it 'positively' (Black and Ong, 1986). However, discomfort, distress and a varied range of mood changes are the experience of many. In a British study, Annette and Graham Scambler (1985) found that no fewer than 82 per cent of their respondents who compiled health diaries, reported at least one distressing symptom (Table 2.6). Negative experiences are reported by women from a range of different cultural backgrounds. The World Health Organization undertook a cross-cultural study of menstruation (Snowden and Christian, 1983) and found that the majority of women in all the cultures investigated reported physical discomfort, and that negative mood changes were widely experienced, also in all cultures (Table 2.7).

Given such widespread experience of difficulties, both physical and psychological, do women perceive menstruation as a condition of health or illness? As discussed earlier in this chapter, for most women 'health' is interpreted as 'feeling good, happy and able to cope'; clearly, these are not sensations always associated with the days of menstruation.

Women's perceptions of menstruation have to be considered in the context of deeply-rooted social and cultural beliefs. Studies reveal that a variety of such beliefs, behavioural restrictions and taboos are associ-

Table 2.6 Menstrual symptoms most frequently defined as distressing either before or during period or both

Symptom	Percentage reporting as distressing
Irritability	49
Pain	30
Fatigue ⎱ Moods ⎰	28
Swelling	27
Headache	25
Depression	24
Weight gain	22
Backache	20
Lowered performance	19
Tension ⎱ Anxiety ⎰	18
Avoidance of social activity	16

Source: Scambler and Scambler, 1985, p. 1066.

Table 2.7 Percentages of respondents experiencing physical discomfort and mood changes prior to or during menstruation

Country	Physical discomfort	Mood changes
Egypt	58	42
India (Hindu, high caste)	58	44
India (Hindu, low caste)	55	40
Indonesia (Javanese)	65	34
Indonesia (Sundanese)	70	23
Jamaica	61	42
Korea	53	52
Mexico	51	38
Pakistan Punjab	50	39
Phillipines	62	48
UK	57	71
Yugoslavia (non-Muslim)	60	65
Yugoslavia (Muslim)	69	73

Source: Snowden and Christian, 1983.

ated with menstruation in widely different societies. Thus, for example, the WHO survey showed that the vast majority of women in all cultures (except in the UK) considered menstruation as 'dirty', and that a variety of religious and cultural demands and customs governed the behaviour of menstruating women such as avoiding cooking (Hindu women in India and women in Jamaica) and not visiting friends (Egypt, India, Jamaica and Yugoslavia). In England, only a generation or two before, strong beliefs about the uncleanliness of menstruating women were held: according to Jeremy Seabrook's account of those times (Seabrook, 1986, p. 203),

> Meat handled by a menstruous woman would go bad. During the last war, the family was scandalised by the fact that my mother looked after a butcher's shop unaided by any male, and for this reason custom diminished appreciably. For many years no member of the family would go to the Co-op because 'all of them gals handlin' the meat when they're like that . . .

In contemporary Western societies, social arrangements surrounding menstruation remain strongly prescriptive: it is for the most part viewed negatively, something to keep hidden and not mentioned in public. Some writers apply the term 'taboo' to the social arrangements and customs surrounding menstruation. Sophie Laws in her interesting and perceptive analysis argues that 'taboo' is inappropriate and 'etiquette' is a better term (Laws, 1985). The notion of taboo implies a consensus of attitudes, whereas here inconsistencies and conflicting views abound; 'taboo' also hides the sexist nature of the attitudes and the power arrangements which make current social prescriptions possible. The subject of menstruation is not 'unmentionable', it is very often discussed in private. Indeed, Sophie Laws' study shows that in exclusively male groups it is referred to frequently.

Menstrual etiquette demands that women (Laws, 1985, p. 16)

> may not make men aware of the existence of menstruation . . . not as a matter of course refer to their own periods in public, feeling a sense of embarrassment or even shame at the thought of doing so.

Although few women perceive menstruation as an illness, their behaviour regarding it resembles that of persons having a stigmatized disease. Sophie Laws argues (Laws, 1985, p. 16) that

> these feelings have often been discussed as though they were spontaneous, springing from something in the woman's own mind,

whereas such feelings result from fear of ridicule by men. According to the study of the Scamblers (1985), only a quarter of the women accepted menstruation as 'normal' or as 'part of life's process' and few regarded it as 'healthy'.

Experiences of discomfort are made worse by the perceived need to conceal them and to pretend that they do not exist. In the workplace, women very rarely mention menstrual pain or mood changes, not only because etiquette forbids, but also because of fears that they will be regarded as unreliable employees by male colleagues and bosses. It is considered wiser to carry on without complaint and to put forward other reasons if sickness absence cannot be avoided. Male respondents, in Sophie Laws' study, demonstrated that such fears are justified: they talked about women being moody, bad tempered and unreliable and mentioned 'the time of the month' when referring to behaviour of which they disapproved. Male interviewees also said that women 'use' menstruation to 'get out of things' or 'to exert control' (Laws, 1985, p. 20).

Thus, menstruation is perceived as an ambiguous mixture of health and illness. It fits into the category of 'health problems which are not real illnesses' and as such is surrounded by uncertainties as to socially approved forms of behaviour.

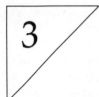

The experience of sickness

Illness behaviour and gender

Research on lay perceptions and explanations has often been conducted with a view to learning about behaviour: health beliefs, notions
of illness and ideas about illness causation all contribute to health and
illness behaviour.

The term 'illness behaviour' has been used by writers since David
Mechanic pointed out in 1962 that systematic variations are to be found
in the ways people perceive, evaluate and act with respect to health
and illness. According to Mechanic's more recent definition (Mechanic,
1982, p. 1)

> illness behaviour describes the manner in which persons monitor
> their bodies, define and interpret their symptoms, take remedial
> actions, and utilize the health-care system.

Following Mechanic, many sociologists demonstrated that variations
in illness behaviour are both systematic and considerable and that
class, gender and culture, among other factors, have a major influence
on the ways individuals act in matters of health. Research on illness
behaviour and gender differences therein has been extensive, but on
the whole rather unsatisfactory. Two decades after Mechanic drew
attention to variations in behaviour, Juanna Clarke (1983) found it
impossible clearly to describe and account for differences in the illness
experiences of women and men; she argued, correctly, that concepts of
health and illness lack clarity and that studying the empirical reality is
beset by methodological problems.

The study of gender differences in illness behaviour suffers from many of the methodological problems that affect the whole field of sociological research. Large-scale surveys provide much interesting but rather generalized information about patterns of behaviour in populations; the subjective meanings and interpretations given by individuals to the events in their lives and to the actions they take, tend to be left unexplored. On the other hand, small-scale studies, specifically designed to explore individuals' subjective understanding of life events, and conducted on particular, well defined, small groups (for example, White working-class women in traditional communities in Scotland, or middle-class White women in California) in isolation from other studies, often leave sociologists with a number of interesting but unrelated and even contradictory insights and clues to behaviour, without providing them with an overall picture.

Certainly there are good grounds for arguing the existence of gender differences in health and illness behaviour. In the first place, women's experiences of pregnancy and childbirth, menstruation and menopause, cause them to think about their bodies, their bodily sensations, and their health in ways foreign to the thinking of men, rendering it unlikely that their illness behaviour would not differ. Secondly, socialization for gender roles during childhood, i.e. learning what constitutes socially approved 'feminine' and 'masculine' behaviour, and what does not, influences the thinking of adults of both sexes as to the suitability of their actions in any given situation; thus health and illness behaviour become gender-specific. Thirdly, structural differences in the lives of men and women (for example, differential experiences in work, unemployment and life-style) and different ways of relating to other people, all have a bearing on their behaviour in health and illness. Lastly, the morbidity rates of men and women are different (see Chapter 1). Behaviour variables of social class and ethnic origin cut across gender differences but information on the interplay of these variables with gender is very scanty.

The reader of the numerous research studies related to the health and illness behaviour of women, becomes aware of two contradictory social expectations. Women are expected to display traits of modesty, frailty and sensitivity, signalling to men that they will be uncompetitive, submissive to them, and likely to make good wives! But these same women are expected to be strong enough to bear and rear children, do all the domestic work, and assume responsibility for the family's health and happiness. The second set of expectations requires robust good health and is at odds with the first which postulates a condition akin to sickliness. Faced with these conflicting 'rules', women have each to develop a strategy for playing the 'health game'.

If one thing is said more than another about gender differences in health and illness behaviour it is that women are more likely than men to be concerned about issues of health and illness and to notice health-related problems in themselves, their children and their spouses. It is not surprising that women have more awareness and knowledge of these matters; menses, reproductive experiences and hormonal changes, stimulate interest, put women in contact with medical services, and form the subject of many woman-to-woman discussions. Moreover, in contemporary Western societies, besides responsibility for the diet and rude health of the family, the care of the young, and of old and disabled family members, is regarded as the province of women (Graham, 1984), obliging them to take more interest in these 'duties' and to equip themselves with more relative information. Whether women develop an interest in health and illness topics because of their biology, or because of social expectations (frequently both) it is the case that, compared to men, they read more articles, watch more television programmes, and listen to more radio broadcasts, on health matters, so adding to their knowledge and expertise. But such media presentations, backed up by advertisements, all too often reinforce the view that it is the woman's job to watch over the health of the family – a duty which is held to include everything from preparing the meals, sanitizing the toilets, and ensuring that the children brush their teeth.

That the mass media reaffirms society's traditional view of women's responsibilities and duties has been illustrated with many examples by Anne Karpf in her study (Karpf, 1988, p. 69) of British television's reporting of health and medicine.

> Health promotion literature and look-after-yourself programmes are generally aimed at women, though they often address men's health. Women are meant to wrestle not only with their own flab, but his too. *Flora* margarine ads . . . cajoled women to get their man using *Flora* instead of butter to trim his waistband and preserve his heart . . .

How do women distinguish between health and illness in themselves and others? Picking up problems in children and husbands usually begins with noticing a change from what was, until then, their normal condition. Such change may be in appetite, mood, vitality or physical appearance (Robinson, 1971). It has been noted that mothers are very skilful in observing changes in the appearance or behaviour of their babies and older children (Spencer, 1984). A different 'look in the baby's eyes' can alert a mother to problems. It is notoriously difficult, however, to notice early manifestations of mental illness in the family (Yarrow, 1955), not only because indications may be extremely varied but also because wives resist the very concept (Miles, 1987).

Noticing changes in oneself is far from straightforward: frequently symptoms fluctuate, pains come and go, and even people who think themselves knowledgeable about health matters lack certainty as to the level of symptom experience that should be heeded. The dual expectation that women should be both robust and frail adds to the difficulty. Moreover, noticing health problems in children or husband prompts positive action to deal with those problems; a personal problem faces one with the more difficult decisions of first, whether to acknowledge it, and second whether to report it, and to whom.

Several studies show that women, when asked by interviewers or health professionals, report more symptoms than do men. During interviews with a sample of 1400 adults, Karen Dunnell and Ann Cartwright (1972) asked them to list the symptoms they experienced during the two-week period prior to the interviews. There was a substantial difference between patterns of symptom reporting by women and by men at all ages over 24: women consistently listed more symptoms than did the men. This disparity can be regarded as indicating:

(a) that women have more symptoms;
(b) that women more readily recognize symptoms because they are better informed about health problems;
(c) that they are more willing to acknowledge and report their problems.

One of the explanations advanced to account for women's greater acceptance of health problems is that gender socialization induces them to behave as the 'weaker sex'. At an early age girls learn that femininity and frailty are compatible, even synonymous, and that it is acceptable for them to express openly sensations of pain and discomfort, unlike boys for whom it is 'unmanly' to fuss. Thus, women in Western societies allow themselves to take notice of symptoms causing discomfort and report them more readily than do men.

In an early study, in which information was obtained from children, Mechanic (1968) found evidence of sex-role socialization in respect of health and illness. He noted that boys were more likely than girls to feel that they have to behave in a stoical manner and bear pain bravely; boys expected their mothers to be less brave than their fathers.

The medical profession has traditionally reinforced this early gender socialization by regarding women biologically as the weaker sex, their lives governed by their reproductive system which renders them prone to more than their fair share of health problems. In their examination of medical textbooks of the last 150 years, Barbara Ehrenreich and Deidre English (1979, p. 110) showed that the theories which guided the doctor's practice from the late nineteenth century to the early twentieth century held that women's normal state was to be sick. This was not advanced as an empirical observation, but as physiological fact.

Thus female frailty was stressed by doctors and emphasized by patterns of values which held that women are the weaker sex.

It is an important and deeply-rooted characteristic of current Western social values that feminine traits, in this case interest in and sensitivity to health issues, are less valued than masculine traits which are the antithesis thereof.

To explain differential illness behaviour in terms of gender socialization is somewhat unsatisfactory, not least because to do so fails to take account of class differences in behaviour. Many of the past studies on women's symptom reporting, and on women's interest in health issues, neglected to differentiate between patterns of middle-class and working-class women, but nevertheless there are indications of differences. Ehrenreich and English noted that doctors in the past regarded only their middle-class female patients as 'biologically weak', encouraging them to pay attention to their complaints; working class women they regarded as 'biologically strong' and these were encouraged to ignore their complaints and to continue working. Current studies also point to differences in doctors' behaviour and advice to middle- and working-class patients. There is also evidence that gender socialization and cultural norms are patterned according to social class. In a study by Cornwell (1984), working-class women spoke strongly against the 'moaners' in their groups.

Becoming aware of a symptom and regarding it as serious depends a great deal on its disruptive potential: the same symptom may be seen as threatening or trivial according to the social context in which it occurs. If a pain or some other distressful symptom disrupts important social roles, it will quickly be noticed and regarded as serious. In this way, the evaluation of symptoms is directly linked to the social structure which shapes the activities, responsibilities and obligations of individuals. For example, severe low back pain, which afflicts many women, is especially disruptive for those who have to care for disabled, sick, or elderly family members impairing, as it does, their ability to lift and carry. Not only the women so affected but their families and doctors are likely to regard such pain as serious. Symptoms of agoraphobia (fear of public places) may not greatly threaten the social functioning of the full-time housewife and may consequently be evaluated by her and her husband as unimportant, indeed confirming the home as her proper sphere of activity.

Of course, life-threatening symptoms are taken seriously whether immediately disruptive or not; but a great deal of pain, discomfort and distress is evaluated according to perceived social responsibilities and obligations which are seldom questioned in this context.

Seeking medical help

If symptoms noted in oneself do not soon disappear, a decision has to be made as to what action should be taken. There are several possibilities: advice can be sought from friends and relatives, home remedies or over-the-counter medicines can be tried, or professional experts approached.

In Western societies, especially during the last 40 years, people have increasingly turned to doctors with their health-related problems: however, advice-seeking from the lay group and from professionals other than doctors and the use of unprescribed remedies, have not declined in popularity. The various actions that people take are not necessarily sequential, nor are they mutually exclusive. Someone may consult friends, pharmacists and doctors in combination or as alternatives, and may use medicines prescribed by doctors while having recourse to home remedies. The importance attached to these possible courses of action will differ from one individual to another, according to his or her position in the social structure, and to prevalent social norms.

One of the most frequently demonstrated gender differences in illness behaviour is found in medical consultation rates. In most Western countries, women go to doctors more frequently than do men, the disparity being most marked when the figures for women of child-bearing age are compared with those for men of corresponding age groups. This might seem obvious and it is all the more intriguing to find that examinations for pregnancy and gynaecological problems do not alone account for the difference in consultation rates. It is also the case that for life-threatening diseases there is little between the sexes when it comes to seeking medical help and it therefore follows that consultations for non-life-threatening problems of illness and disability must account for the remaining difference in consultation patterns (Verbrugge, 1982; Waldron, 1983a).

In countries outside Western Europe and North America, the pattern of consultation varies. For example, in Thailand women have the higher rates, whereas in India and Bangladesh men make more use of medical services; in Japan, there has been a striking change from higher medical visit rates for men in the 1950s to higher rates for women in the 1970s (Waldron, 1983b).

Why do women consult doctors more often than do men? In an

attempt to answer this question, three possibilities have been explored by researchers. Firstly, there is the 'differential need' explanation, according to which women have more health-related problems and consequently need more often to consult doctors. Secondly, the 'differential predisposing factors' explanation contains the argument that women's perceptions, attitudes and past experiences, make them more willing to seek medical help; and thirdly, there is the 'differential enabling factors' explanation, according to which women are in a better position to go to the doctor's surgery than are men.

Attempts to examine the 'need' factor, i.e. determining whether women's health is really worse than that of men, lead to a morass of confusion and contradictions. As already discussed, health and illness are socially construed notions which mean different things to different people. Disagreements as to what constitutes illness abound; there may be a consensus as to the 'killer' diseases being 'real' illnesses, but whether alcohol dependency, depression or disabilities following amputation, to name a few, are 'illnesses' or not is a matter for dispute among both lay and professionally-trained people. Moreover, the assumption that there are 'real' illnesses and thus real needs, to which individuals then respond (i.e. the distinction between illness and illness behaviour), rests on the notion that a biophysical reality exists and has primacy over human interpretation. But it can be argued, as Clarke suggests (Clarke, 1983), that

> this is a false dichotomy because human beings are social actors. As such they must continually construct social reality. The physical realm is not separate: it can only be known through social interpretation. From this viewpoint it does not make sense to speak of symptoms except as they are socially constructed.

Methodological problems of determining morbidity (ill health in the population) and the resulting needs, are as great as the conceptual problems. Different researchers use many different indices of illness and of need for medical care; there are contradictions between needs as perceived by the patients, their relatives, and health professionals. Moreover, it is apparent that the state of medical knowledge, the existence or absence of services and of effective treatments as well as issues of access, all influence 'need' and measuring it is a very problematic exercise.

To raise the conceptual and methodological problems of exploring gender-related differences in ill health, is not to deny the possibility of such differences. It is possible that women experience more pain and discomfort than men do but the available conceptual tools are not adequate for clarifying whether differences lie in bodily sensations, or in the socially-constructed meanings attached to them.

In spite of conceptual and methodological problems (and often ignoring their implications) researchers have carried out studies in this area. It is of interest to note that a number of inventories and checklists have been developed to measure people's overall health status, both physical and mental, and studies based on such measures explored the association between health-status and consultation rates. Other researchers also investigated the correlation between perceived symptoms and decisions to go to the doctor (Belloc *et al.*, 1971).

Monica Briscoe (1987) studied the patients of a London general practitioner and found, as expected, that the mean annual number of consultations was higher for women than for men (3.8 and 2.0, respectively). After the exclusion of sex-specific consultations for pregnancy and post-natal examinations, she found that differences between women and men were marked in consultations for acute conditions (the male: female ratio was almost 1:2), and that women were three times as likely to consult for more than one condition. (She also found that men received many more sickness certificates for employment absence than did women.) When she examined the overall health status of her sample, using a physical health inventory and the patients' reports of their experience of symptoms over the previous year, she found that there was no significant association between need and women's consulting behaviour. In other words, women who appeared to be in poorer health overall, consulted the doctors no more than did women who enjoyed better overall health. Thus, the simple proposition that women go to the doctor more than men do because women have more illnesses is not supported by her findings.

Predisposing factors play an important part in decisions to seek medical help. Such factors include general beliefs about health and illness, knowledge and information about symptoms, treatments, and the working of the body, attitudes to the medical profession and to medical knowledge, and interest in health issues. As previously discussed, it has been demonstrated that gender differences in such factors can be marked and it is not surprising to find in women a greater predisposition to turn to doctors than is found in men. Another factor influencing willingness to consult a doctor is that the role of the help-seeker is a dependent and submissive one: the patient seeks help and advice from a doctor who is assumed to have superior knowledge and skills and who is in a position to instruct and give orders. Women are socialized and pressed into accepting the feminine role, which is compatible with the position of a submissive and dependent help-seeker (Chesler, 1972). Accordingly, women are more willing to place themselves into such a position than are men whose gender role prepares them much less for the role of the patient.

Curiously, little attention has been given to the role of the medical profession in predisposing women to seek its help. Doctors actively encourage consultation with particular problems and discourage it with regard to others, it being likely that the gender of the patient influences the doctor's attitude. A woman's past experience with doctors will bear on her future decisions when she thinks that she needs medical advice. In Britain, where most people are registered with a general practitioner, women know their doctors and know when to seek their help and when there is little point in so doing. In their study of women and menstruation, Annette and Graham Scambler (1985) noted that a third of their sample had consulted their doctors on this matter during the year prior to the research. Many of those who did not go to the doctor during this period experienced a great deal of menstrual distress and discomfort, and even regarded menstruation as a health problem. They did not seek medical help, however, because they felt disillusioned with their doctors in this respect. Many of these women said that their doctors were unresponsive, unsympathetic and unable to help, besides which the fact that most of the doctors previously encountered were male, made help-seeking harder, often leading to feelings of 'being let down' (Scambler and Scambler, 1985, p. 1067):

> I don't consult – I haven't bothered again – I don't feel they understand the problem, and it is so hard to explain.

> I would go, but only when it was necessary. Men haven't been through it, so they can't know all about it.

It is possible that in the United States women are more inclined to seek medical help for problems connected with menstruation: indeed, there are estimates that premenstrual tension is currently one of the commonest conditions for which American women consult doctors (Shuttle and Redgrove, 1986). Perhaps greater flexibility in the choice of doctors (at least for those able to pay) has a bearing on this.

The term 'enabling factor' refers to those considerations which either facilitate or hinder help-seeking from doctors ('disenabling factor' might better describe the latter). Some writers have found it convenient to explore such factors within a framework of 'perceived costs' against 'perceived benefits', suggesting that the decision to go to the doctor is arrived at via a process of weighing the pros and cons of such a visit. The 'perceived costs' of a consultation might be financial, or be seen in terms of lost time, anticipated embarrassment or unpleasantness, difficulty of access, etc., while the 'perceived benefits' might include the obtainment of treatment, relief from pain, receipt of a certificate authorizing absence from work, a prescription for sleeping pills and plain reassurance.

Is there anything, peculiar to the lives of women, which reduces the cost, or increases the benefit, of a visit to the doctor, and so might provide some explanation of their more frequent consultations? The arguments are contradictory and the balance of the evidence shows that this is not the case. One of the arguments is that the very many women who do not 'go out to work' have more time, and greater flexibility in organizing their affairs, than have either men or women in outside employment, thus making it easier for them to arrange often time-consuming visits to their doctors. However, Oakley's studies on housework showed that the alleged flexibility is not as great as previously assumed, and (as several writers have pointed out) that the presence of young children at home, and the needs of schoolchildren, make considerable demands on time and reduce flexibility (Oakley, 1974). Indeed, Nathanson (1975), argued that women with heavy family commitments find it difficult to make time to see the doctor and that they therefore look for alternative solutions.

Several studies have investigated the effects of employment, and of the presence of children, on consultation rates. Thus, Monica Briscoe (1987) found, in her London sample, that employment was not a significant factor, but that parental roles were associated with higher rates for both women and men. In the United States, Janet Meininger (1986), on the basis of a study with a White, working-class sample, showed likewise, that employment status had no meaningful effect on consultation rates of either women or men. Interestingly, Meininger also found that presence of children in the home had a significant effect on the consultation rates of men. She accounted for this by hypothesizing that the presence of children may reinforce the traditional bread-winning role of men, leading them to watch their health rather more carefully than is the case of men without children. One might further conjecture that greater responsibilities, financial pressures, crying babies, sleepless nights, and tired wives are all stress factors tending to higher illness rates.

There are many other factors which may facilitate or hinder medical help-seeking. Even when people do not have to pay for consultations, financial, economic and practical difficulties abound. The important resources of time and money greatly influence going to the doctor; for example, studies show that mothers of young children find it difficult to visit clinics or surgeries where lengthy journeys are involved, as neither leaving children at home, nor taking them along is practicable. Hilary Graham found that pregnant mothers were less able to attend clinics for antenatal care where services were provided centrally at hospitals rather than in local doctors' surgeries (Graham, 1984).

Even so, transport to and from surgeries can present problems. Although the majority of households in Britain and in the United States have the use of a car, the women have far less access to it than the men. Many more men have driving licences and often, men have first claim on the car for travel to work.

The many financial and practical constraints which exist are all likely to be greater for women who are single parents, rendering them less able than other mothers to visit doctors' surgeries.

Why then do women have higher rates of medical consultation? Examining the recorded reasons for consultations, it seems that the main gender difference is in the seeking of help for psychological, emotional and vague but disquieting physical problems – women being the more likely to consult doctors for such reasons.

According to Waldron, in the United States, women's visits to doctors for psychological and mental symptoms, social counselling and weight gain is far in excess of similar consultations by men (Waldron, 1983a) while in Britain and elsewhere in Western Europe, estimates of female:male ratios in consultations for neurotic and psycho-social problems vary between 2:1 and 4:1 (Weissman and Klerman, 1977). Monica Briscoe's study of gender differences in consultation rates also showed that (Briscoe, 1987, p. 509)

the most striking difference between the sexes concerned the relationship between consultation rates and psychological help-seeking. Here there was a significant positive relationship for the women and an equally significant negative relationship among the men, so that high consultation rates were associated with willingness to seek psychiatric help among the women, and un-willingness among the men.

It is possible then that many women, as a result of socialization, current social norms and doctors' attitudes ('predisposing factors' discussed earlier), allow themselves to seek help for emotional problems, whereas many men may be discouraged from doing so.

Some caution is necessary here; the basis of most studies on reasons for consultation is the diagnosis made and recorded by doctors. But diagnosis is not a 'neutral', 'objective' or 'value-free' decision: the patient's gender could influence diagnosis. Doctors may record psychological and emotional problems as reasons for consultations more readily for female than for male patients.

The consequences of consulting for emotional problems (whether so described by the patient, or seen by the doctor in this light) are not entirely beneficial for women. On the one hand they gain access to whatever help and treatment is available; on the other, the negative stereotyping of the 'sickly and neurotic woman' gains credence.

Of course, gender is not alone in influencing help-seeking from doctors. Social class background and ethnic origin have bearings on medical help-seeking. Many British studies have shown that patterns of consultation are different for middle and for working-class families, although the nature of the difference remains rather elusive. Very few studies have explored the interplay of gender and class in this field. Janet Meininger (1986) had the interesting finding that in the United States, women of lower social classes were more likely to seek medical help than were middle-class women. She thought it possible that middle-class women have more access to other forms of help and are better able to seek advice from alternative sources. In Britain, Hilary Homans (1985) noted that middle-class women were more likely than working-class women to turn to doctors as a first resort with discomforts of pregnancy. She also showed that Asian women (from Punjab and Gujerat) living in Britain are less likely than White women to go to doctors with complaints during pregnancy, but that this may be changing as other sources of help (family ties) are breaking down. The difficulties experienced by Black women and Hispanic women seeking help from White doctors in Britain and in the United States have been frequently demonstrated: adverse experiences may well result in their becoming reluctant seekers of help. It seems clear that cultural norms, past experiences with doctors, and the existence of alternative help sources, are more influential factors on medical help-seeking than the doctors' actual ability to help to cure the symptoms.

Restoration of health without doctors

The onset of a health problem does not invariably result in a visit to the doctor; on the contrary, by far the greater part of symptom experience does not so result. It has been estimated that only 1 in 10 (some would say 1 in 30) symptoms are taken to the doctor.

What other actions do people take in response to health problems? One option is to do nothing: to wait, to ignore the problem in the hope that it will prove temporary and insignificant. This is a common response to conditions which are familiar and seem minor, such as coughs, colds and headaches. There is also a temptation to ignore symptoms which might indicate a fearful, frightening or stigmatizing disease. Thus, for example, hallucinations, or a lump on the breast will be disregarded, at least for a while, because madness, or cancer, is too frightening to contemplate.

Another reason for not taking action is that help-seeking and medicine-taking for a particular problem are frowned upon by the social group of the sufferer. The views of the immediate social group regarding the appropriate evaluation of symptoms, and responses to them, are very important. Freidson drew attention to the importance of obtaining views from the lay circle on individual decision-making: lay

consultations regarding health problems he described as the 'lay referral' system, arguing that discussions about specific problems usually
result in some advice being given by friends and relatives as to the
meaning of the problem and the best way of dealing with it. Accordingly, such advice contains an implicit diagnosis of the problem and
either a 'referral', i.e. a prescription as to the best kind of helper to
consult or a consensus that no action is necessary (Freidson, 1975a).

Women very often discuss health matters with other women and this
process of advice-giving and advice-seeking, with its implicit diagnosis
and prescription, influences illness behaviour. For example, women
suffering from depression frequently report having talked to other
women about feeling 'low', 'not coping', or sleeplessness, before decid-
ing to go to the doctor (Miles, 1988). Some of them were advised that
the doctor should be consulted, while others were told to 'snap out of
it' and 'not to make too much of it'. The nature of the advice usually
depended on whether or not the person consulted had experienced
similar problems herself; but interestingly women with depression had
nearly always taken the advice of their lay group initially, and tried to
ignore the problem, or consulted the doctor, according to that advice.
For these women, lay advice was accepted, not because they thought
their lay group particularly well informed and competent to give it, but
because it indicated the behaviour that was approved by the group in
the particular situation. Acting in line with lay advice gave confidence
that social disapproval would not follow: thus one young mother said
(Miles, 1988, p. 97):

> At the beginning I was feeling very low, I didn't want to go
> anywhere, didn't want to eat. I could hardly face the day when
> I woke up in the morning. I told my sister about it, and my
> neighbours, when we had the children's party . . . they all said I
> will feel better and not to give in . . . they said I mustn't start to
> take pills. I didn't go to my doctor, didn't want them to laugh at
> me, I thought I'd try to snap out of it.

A different sort of advice was given to a middle-aged woman, experiencing symptoms which she thought may be due to the menopause, who said (Miles, 1988, p. 97):

> I talked it over with them [two women friends] and also asked
> somebody I work with, a women who is about my age, and they
> told me to go to the doctor. I was embarrassed, didn't want to
> waste the doctor's time, but when everybody told me to go, I
> thought I would.

Thus, lay referral delayed the seeking of medical advice in the one case
and prompted it in other.

Lay advice is often sought and offered concerning another possible response to symptoms – a change in life-style (e.g. eating habits). Lay discussion is specially frequent when health problems relate to the menses, pregnancy and associated matters.

Many changes in life-style are advocated and tried: taking more exercise, eating at different times, resting more or less, etc. Such measures are attractive partly because they can all be tried without seeking expert advice. The World Health Organization's survey on menstruation found that increased rest and reduction of work were very usual responses to menstrual pain: in the U.K., 22 per cent of women reported resting more than usual during menstruation. Pregnant women often change eating times and alter their diet to avoid flatulence and indigestion.

There is evidence to indicate that many people in Britain and the United States rely on so called 'folk medicine' (or traditional medicine) and certainly there is a current revival of interest in these remedies, especially among women (Chamberlain, 1981). Minor illnesses and discomforts during the 'natural' biological processes are treated by many women in this way. Hilary Homans (1985) found that in her sample the majority of Asian women living in Britain (mostly of Punjabi origin) used traditional remedies for discomforts of pregnancy (73 per cent) which they usually learnt from older female relatives. White British women in the same study were less likely to have relevant knowledge, but even among them, 35 per cent knew and used 'folk' remedies (milk, lemonade, *Polo*, roughage in the diet, almonds, ginger and many other remedies are tried for stomach problems in pregnancy). Among White British women the use of folk remedies is closely related to class; past studies have demonstrated that working-class women, much more than middle-class women, incline to these remedies. However, the gulf between them may be narrowing with the proliferation of health-food shops, advocating herbal and 'natural' remedies and food, which are increasingly patronized by middle-class women.

Treating ailments with medicines obtained from drugstores, pharmacists and supermarkets, is also very popular. In their survey of medicine-taking, Karen Dunnel and Ann Cartwright (1972) noted that women were specially large consumers of over-the-counter, self-prescribed, medicines. Indeed, three-quarters of the women had taken some such medicine during the fortnight before they were interviewed as compared to three-fifths of the men. Apparently the women did not take more medicines merely because they had more symptoms, but rather were more likely to take medicines for their symptoms. Trying to account for their findings, Dunnell and Cartwright (1972, pp. 21–22) considered some practical issues:

One possible explanation for women's higher consumption of non-prescribed medicines is that they generally take responsibility for the family shopping. They will therefore be exposed to the display and advertising of remedies in shops. This may make them more likely to buy over-the-counter medicines for their symptoms. In addition, women spend more time than men in the home, and the average household has ten different items of medicine in it. In short, medicines may be more readily available to women and they may more often be made aware of them.

The purchase of manufactured drugs in shops may not, then, depend on medical advice; on the other hand, it may involve the pharmacist, and there are indications that people seek the advice of these specialists about their symptoms and buy drugs on their recommendation. Pharmacists are only one of the groups of professional experts outside the medical profession whose advice is sought; health visitors, community nurses, and many others give advice, as well as the growing number of healers who practise what is called 'alternative' medicine. Indeed, women have contact, at various times, with a range of professional and lay helpers, and it is important to recognize that the 'authorized' medical services are among a variety of help-sources to which an individual may turn, selecting one or more of them to advise about any particular health problem. The wide range of possible responses to symptoms makes for complexity in decision-taking.

Women and the sick role

Being sick is both an individual experience and a social state. Sensations of pain and discomfort, feelings of panic and disorientation, are intensely individual and personal. Indeed, people often find it difficult to explain their sensations and experiences to others, especially to those who lack personal acquaintance with similar symptoms. However, the evaluation of pain and discomfort as part or not of normal health, the attribution of causes to unpleasant bodily sensations, the behaviour considered appropriate to a sick person and the responses of others to the sickness of an individual, are all governed by the culture of a society, and by features of that society's structure, and constitute the social dimension of sickness. The notion of sickness as a social state was formulated very clearly by Freidson (Freidson, 1975a, p. 208):

> In human society, naming something an illness has consequences independent of the biological state of the organism. Consider two men in different societies, both with the same debilitating infec-

tion: in one case, the man is said to be ill, put to bed, and taken care of by others; in the other case, he is said to be lazy, and he is abused by others. The course and outcome of the disease may be the same biologically in both cases, but the social interplay between the sick man and others is significantly different. And consider the social consequences of diagnosis behaviour: one diagnosis may lead to 'cure', another diagnosis may lead to death. While disease may be 'there', it is what we, as social beings, think and do about it that determines the content of our lives.

Thus, sociologists are interested in the character of sickness as a social state. An individual, on experiencing pain, discomfort or other indication of the presence of a biological malfunctioning of the body, may, though not necessarily, assume the 'sick-role', i.e. the social role of the sick person. The theoretical concept of the sick role was first developed by Talcott Parsons in a series of papers published during the 1950s (Parsons, 1951; Parsons, 1958), and although criticized by some subsequent writers and elaborated by others, the concept provides a useful framework for discussion. Parsons developed a model for the sick role as part of his critique of the then prevailing conceptualization of illness as a solely biological state and medical concern; he set out to provide a sociological alternative to the dominant medical model. He described certain social expectations and associated sanctions affecting the sick, and defined the sick role in terms of four components:

(i)   sick persons are allowed by society to withdraw from some or all of their social obligations and responsibilities (e.g. work, family duties);
(ii) sick persons are exempted from responsibility for their sickness and no blame is attached to them;
(iii) they have the obligation to define their sickness as undesirable, to wish to get well and return to normal social obligations;
(iv) they must endeavour to seek appropriate help (usually from a physician) and co-operate with professional recommendations and treatment.

This concept of the sick role is of somewhat limited applicability: the assumption is made that the sick person will get better and return to previous social roles, a reasonable enough assumption in cases of acute illness but not for chronic conditions and long-term disabilities. This limitation forms one of the criticisms that has been levelled against Parsons' model; others concern Parsons' apparently exclusive concentration on Western industrial societies and his lack of recognition that even in those societies there exists a diversity of social groups with unequal access to the sick role (according to such variables as socio-economic position and gender), and with a range of social values which govern action in sickness. There is also the criticism that underlying the sick-role model is Parsons' assumption that relationships between doctors and patients are always harmonious, and not, as they sometimes are, contentious (Freidson, 1975b; Bloor and Horobin, 1975).

Despite such reservations the sick role concept has its defenders. Bryan Turner (1987) argued that critics were wrong to allege that Parsons' notion applies only to Western industrial societies; he refers to the issue of withdrawal from social activities on sickness, perhaps the most important part of Parsons' concept, saying that (Turner, 1977, p. 55)

> the sick role as a form of social withdrawal is widespread in human cultures and clearly not peculiar to modern industrial societies. For example, in the Islamic Middle East illness can be a method for legitimating behaviour which deviates from conventional social expectations...

Turner points to anthropological research in the Nile delta, and regarding North-American tribes, which demonstrates that there are in many societies culturally patterned disorders which are social roles and can be regarded essentially as 'sick-roles', although with different kinds of healers being involved in legitimization and with different codes of conduct surrounding withdrawal from social obligations.

Interest in the concept of the sick role is maintained because the notion that there is a social role for the sick person in society is important and because it provides a useful analytical tool in the study of illness behaviour. Part of the usefulness of Parsons' model during the past 30 years has been that it poses questions which inspire researchers to set out and explore the range of answers which would reflect the empirical reality.

Sociologists currently studying the experiences of sick persons are faced with several problem areas, mainly the issue of legitimate access to the sick role, the imputation of responsibility for sickness by the social group to the sick person, and the applicability of the sick role to long-term or permanent conditions and to situations which do not fit clearly into either sickness or health. These problems which are of particular interest for the sickness experiences and behaviour of women are discussed below.

Legitimacy and access

An important and problematic issue in the analysis of the experience of sickness in Western societies concerns the circumstances in which assuming the sick role is possible and appropriate. As said, inherent in the notion of the sick role is withdrawal from daily activities and responsibilities. Indeed, the distinction between experiencing symptoms of illness and occupying the sick role lies in the sick person's discontinuance of usual activities. Not everyone who has an illness assumes the sick role; many people with minor illnesses and some with more major ones, continue with their normal range of activities.

The usual path to the sick role is to claim it: it is for individuals to express their inability to continue normal functioning. This is not invariably so: there are cases when someone is required, although unwilling, to withdraw from social activities, for example when mental illness is attributed to a person who does not accept it, or in cases of alcoholism or when infection may be spread by contact; in such circumstances, social norms may well demand of the affected person that the sick role be adopted.

Some people are quite reluctant to claim the sick role, even while accepting the presence of illness; some are unable to do so, but most are ready enough to withdraw from some or all of their customary activities in the face of sickness and it is with these that Talcott Parsons was chiefly concerned. His analysis of sickness in society was essentially functionalist: he considered social activities in terms of their 'contributions' to the maintenance of the social system. From a functionalist perspective Parsons argued that if a very large number of people abandon their social activities at any one time, society cannot function, or at least severe social strains would be experienced. Therefore, withdrawal from activities through sickness must be regulated. Legitimization of the sick role, and the placing of obligations on the sick person, must be viewed as social control mechanisms.

What exercized Parsons was the consideration that there is, for some people, a positive motivation to assume the sick role. Examples of this abound in research findings of his time and in subsequent studies. Consider, for example, the woman who is looking after her twin mentally handicapped teenage sons, providing constant nursing for them, as well as caring for other, younger children (Miles, 1988); she is chronically tired and life seems a hopeless struggle without respite. A period of sickness, necessitating removal to hospital, would appear as a most welcome relief. Indeed, Claudine Herzlich (1973, p. 114) found that some respondents regarded illness as a liberator (see Chapter 2) describing it in such terms as 'it's a sort of holiday' or 'illness is a kind of rest when you can be free of your everyday burden'. This motivation to escape into the sick role would certainly be very understandable in the case of women who care for disabled or elderly relatives or whose time is taken up by domestic work with only young children as company. Relentless routine, feelings of being trapped with no prospect of relief, might well make an illness episode seem attractive. It is at least possible that a glimmer of such hope influences some women to go to the doctor with symptoms of tiredness, headaches, sleeplessness, backache, etc., which others, in different circumstances, would regard as 'part of life', not necessitating medical intervention.

However, not everyone is so ready to escape into sickness; there are contrary pressures on women which make them less willing to assume the sick role. Studies of mothers and female carers at home tend to show that many women see themselves as indispensable. Indeed, the feeling that they are so is very important, as it constitutes one of the few positive and pleasurable rewards for putting up with harsh conditions. To conceive of oneself as indispensable to the family welfare is likely to influence women against claiming the sick role, even when painful symptoms are present.

Reluctance to assume the sick role is consistent with another pattern found by Herzlich among French respondents, some of whom saw illness as destructive and intolerable; typically this thinking characterized those who saw themselves as indispensable.

Feelings of being all-important to their young children or to disabled and elderly relatives are frequently grounded in stark reality: there is literally no one else who could or would replace the mother or carer. For example, studies of one-parent families show the severe problems that arise when the parent is ill; single mothers are revealed as reluctant to go to the doctor because medical advice may involve giving up activities with no one available to take over (Marsden, 1973; Evason, 1980). Mothers of severely handicapped children are in a similar situation (Baldwin and Glendinning, 1983). Hilary Graham argued that (Graham, 1984, p. 159)

> while a mother is quick to identify and respond to symptoms of illness and disability in others, she appears less assiduous in monitoring her own health. Her role in caring for others appears to blunt her sensitivity to her own needs. Being ill makes it difficult for individuals to maintain their normal roles and responsibilities: since the mother's roles and responsibilities are particularly indispensable, mothers are reluctant to be ill.

The social class position of women greatly influences behaviour when it comes to claiming the sick role. A much quoted early study illustrated the feelings of many women of the poorer classes in the United States (Koos, 1954, p. 30):

> I wish I knew what you mean by being sick. Sometimes I felt so bad I could curl up and die, but I had to go on because of the kids who have to be taken care of and besides, we didn't have the

money to spend for the doctor. How could I be sick? Some people can be sick any time with anything, but most of us can't be sick, even when we need to be.

Contemporary confirmation is contained in the studies of working class women by Pill and Stott (1982), in South Wales, and by Jocelyn Cornwell (1984), in London. The former noted that constraints on adopting the sick role were clearly recognized by three-quarters of their interviewees. Mothers would remark (1982, p. 49) 'of course, I hardly ever go to the doctor', or 'I only go for myself when it is absolutely necessary' while taking the view that the doctor should be seen immediately when problems arose with their children. Cornwell (Cornwell, 1984, p. 141) quoted a woman suffering from a severe form of anaemia who said:

I used to be like an old-age pensioner walking along and all of a sudden everything used to go round. I was walking along and everything used to go black and all the lights used to come before my eyes.

Nevertheless, she carried on.

Of course, going to the doctor is not synonymous with claiming the sick role; on the contrary, many women seek help in order to forestall possible withdrawal from essential duties.

Thus, although the way into the sick role is to claim it, not everyone is equally able to avail themselves of the opportunity to do so, due to a variety of constraints. For women, pressure stemming from the needs of the family can restrict access to the sick role, social class being the underlying factor.

The attitudes of the immediate social group will also greatly influence the taking of a decision to suspend normal functioning. Assumption of the sick role is far more approved of and encouraged in some social settings than in others. The working-class mothers in Wales, interviewed by Pill and Stott, who said that to take the children to the doctor on perceiving a symptom is right, but to present one's own symptoms promptly was not, indicated the norms of their social group in which social approval was accorded to women who 'keep going' even when experiencing discomfort. The authors noted that (Pill and Stott, 1982, p. 50)

moral opprobrium was heaped on those women who were deemed to be too ready to think they were ill and to seek the advantages of the sick role when the appropriate behaviour was seen as 'not giving in' and 'fighting it off' or by 'keeping going and working it off'.

Similar attitudes among working-class people in East London were revealed by Jocelyn Cornwell (1984). Women whom she interviewed did not like to appear to others as 'moaners' and claiming the sick role would seem like 'giving in'.

By contrast, attitudes encouraging women to show weakness, to complain and to claim the sick role quite readily, may appear more amongst middle-class women; for example, Kadushin (1968) showed that in social circles such as entertaining, advertising, arts, people are more ready to claim the sick role for emotional problems.

Women working in paid employment also experience pressure not to claim the sick role too readily: their absence from work through sickness tends to confirm in male colleagues and bosses their stereotypical view of women as the weaker sex, frequently ailing and unreliable as workers.

Not enough is known yet about the cultural norms of ethnic minority groups in Western countries, and there is also a paucity of cross-cultural research on illness behaviour. The available studies indicate a wealth of interesting information, and suggest the need for more research. For example, the World Health Organization's cross-cultural study showed patterns of adopting the sick role as a response to menstruation in different cultures. In some countries surveyed (Mexico, Yugoslavia and the U.K.), urban women were more likely to adopt the sick role than rural women. In many countries the content of the culture determined action: Indian women withdrew from their usual activities, but this was due to the notion of menstrual pollution (although the effect was the same as adoption of the sick role), while in Korea it was important to women to keep menstruation a secret and they were reluctant to adopt the sick role for fear of drawing attention to their condition (Snowden and Christian, 1983).

Claiming the sick role is only the beginning of the process of becoming a legitimate occupier of the role: usually, it is not enough for someone to announce 'I am sick' and thereupon to discontinue all obligations and tasks. What is necessary for legitimate assumption of the sick role is the acceptance of the claim by a person's family, colleagues, employers and friends, i.e. the immediate social group. If these people don't accept that the claim to sickness is justified, disapproval and blame follows, and instead of being regarded as sick, the person making the claim is seen as lazy, a malingerer, or a 'moaner'.

Social groups, therefore, vary in their readiness to accord the sick role. However, not only prevailing norms but also the nature of the complaint influence the members of these groups in according the sick role. In some cases the complainer of illness will be seen as obviously genuine, but in other instances the social group may be undecided as to the validity of the claim to be ill; they will then need independent expert advice. In contemporary Western societies the doctors are regarded as experts in the field of diseases and function as legitimizing agents: usually a person is accepted by the social group as legitimately occupying the sick role if a medical practitioner confirms the presence of a disease requiring withdrawal from activities.

The doctor's legitimizing function is an important feature of the sick-role model as developed by Talcott Parsons. However, Parsons assumed that doctors make decisions concerning the validation of sickness claims on the basis of 'universalistic' norms, i.e. that only the characteristics of the disease influence their decisions, the characteristics of the patients do not, all being treated alike. This assumption is not borne out by empirical research; for example, it was shown that in Britain, doctors' treatment of patients differs significantly according to the social class of the patient (Cartwright and O'Brien, 1976), and a classic ethnographic study conducted in the United States by Sudnow (1967) showed that doctors' responses varied according to the age and presumed moral character of the patient.

There are, also, important gender variations in doctors' judgements: female and male patients do not necessarily have the same chance of obtaining legitimization of their sickness claims. Research findings are contradictory, possibly reflecting the contradictory pressures on doctors and their ambivalent attitudes to women patients. Doctors, most of whom are male (this is changing, but slowly), tend to hold male-orientated views of women and their problems: the stereotype of the weak, complaining, neurotic woman repeatedly appears in views expressed by doctors. Complaints of female patients can be discussed and devalued, as being 'only in the mind', or 'imaginary', due to their having 'too little to occupy them'. Thus, severe pain during menstruation, and symptoms of the menopause, will be dismissed as 'psychosomatic' (Lennane and Lennane, 1973): female sufferers from migraine may well be treated as badly adjusted women (Macintyre and Oldman, 1977).

The subject of doctors' attitudes to and treatment of female patients is discussed in more detail in the chapter concerned with doctor–patient relationships (Chapter 6). Here, it is sufficient to note that besides gender-related influences on women's right to the sick role, there is evidence that women, in a range of situations, find difficulty in obtaining validation of their complaints from doctors.

Difficulties experienced in claiming the sick role are compounded when the social group itself is unsure. Patient, doctor and friends, will all agree that the sick role is appropriate after major surgery or in the presence of an infectious disease; the situation is not so clear with regard to some other conditions and many 'grey areas' exist. Lack of consensus is typical in cases of anxiety, agoraphobia, anorexia and depression, known to doctors as 'minor psychiatric' conditions, and which mainly affect women. The medical profession is uncertain about these problems, some physicians arguing that they constitute genuine illnesses, needing specialist treatment and in serious cases even admission to hospital, while other doctors are of the opinion that the sufferers should 'pull themselves together' and carry on without treatment or recourse to the sick role. Frequently the social group, the family, friends and colleagues, of the depressed, agoraphobic or anorexic woman will incline to the latter view. Even in cases where the doctor wishes to legitimize the sick role, the lay group may be unwilling to agree. A recent study of women diagnosed as 'neurotic' and receiving treatment by psychiatrists, revealed that husbands were reluctant to regard their wives' depression as 'illness' and to accord them the sick role, even when the wives were demonstrably unable to perform their usual tasks and had to withdraw from family obligations just as surely as if they were physically ill (Miles, 1988). Social disapproval follows such lack of acceptance by the group: some women struggling with depression and not able to get up in the morning were labelled as malingerers, in spite of medical validation of their depression as sickness. Thus, one woman said (p. 107)

I used to become exhausted very quickly and quite a few relatives insinuated that I was lazy for sitting down a lot.

This woman was later admitted to the psychiatric department of her local hospital, a clear indication that in the view of doctors the sick role was appropriate and legitimate, but her family and friends continued to question the genuineness of her illness. The fact that it is usually psychiatrists who confirm such conditions and prescribe treatment tends to increase uncertainties and disapproval. Many people are dubious about psychiatrists and unsure about their diagnoses; as legitimizers of illness, psychiatrists are in a far from clear position and their verdicts are more likely to be questioned than are those of physicians.

Responsibility, blame and guilt

An integral part of the sick role is society's acceptance that sick persons are not responsible for their condition, did not bring it about and could not have avoided it. If professionals or lay social groups impute responsibility to sick persons for their sickness, much less sympathy, and assistance is accorded them, rather they meet with social disapproval. Here, again, the psychiatric illnesses, especially those of women, are illustrative of the sorts of condition for which the social group charges responsibility to the sufferer. The view is widely held that physical illness hits people indiscriminately; anyone may become ill, because illness is thought to derive from external agents and no blame is attributable. On the other hand, mental disturbance is often attributed to weakness or character defects and responsibility is imputed (Miles, 1987). Blame attaches even more readily if the complainant is a woman: depression, anxiety, agoraphobia and other problems, which affect women more than men, are widely regarded as signs of weakness, internally induced, which women should not succumb to, but 'shrug off', or ignore. Long periods of depression frequently provoke the comment 'she should pull herself together', implying that the sufferer has brought her problems upon herself and holds the key to recovery in her own hands. Underlying the imputation of blame is the general view of women as weak and complaining, a view held by professionals and lay people alike.

Male sufferers from depression and anxiety, much fewer in numbers, gain greater credibility from doctors and relatives: causes are thought likely to be located in work-related problems for which a man is not blameable; men are regarded as being less likely than women to succumb to problems (Miles, 1988).

Of course, there are cases of physical illness where blame is accorded to the victim of it, for instance when the question of neglect enters the calculation. Neglect of the precautions and care deemed by the social group to be adequate (for example, failure to vaccinate) or neglect of warning signs resulting in more serious illness, are considered blameworthy. The heavy smoker who develops lung cancer will earn censure as well as sympathy, the injuries sustained by a drunken driver will meet with condemnation from the social group, the more so if others also are hurt.

Jocelyn Cornwell (1984) in her study of working-class families in East London quoted examples of people being blamed for neglecting illness. Interviewing the relatives of a certain Nellie about her ill-health, she found (p. 152) that they 'believed that it was caused by her attitude towards herself and that it was therefore something that could be avoided, for which therefore she was to blame'. According to these relatives (p. 153),

> she's always been ill, but it's her own bloody fault, she can't be bothered to go to the doctor's. She hasn't even got to go to the doctor's, she's on the 'phone. She's only got to 'phone over for the doctor to come over to her, but she can't be bothered. She don't want to go to a hospital because she's frightened she'll never come out, which is ridiculous, because you don't have to stay on.

Thus, Nellie's relatives accorded blame and lack of sympathy followed.

It does not always follow that social disapproval and lack of sympathy are consequent upon the laying of blame. It can happen that certain individuals have become so disliked or caused such exasperation among their associates, that friends and relatives are ready to award blame almost regardless of the circumstances of the case. One thing is clear – imputing responsibility, according blame, and denying sympathy, constitute a 'package', an inter-related set of responses to the sickness of individuals and the circumstances surrounding that sickness.

Not only lay social groups but health professionals also respond differently to sick people whom they hold responsible for the illness than they do to those seen as blameless. Sudnow's study (1967) was conducted at a hospital emergency unit in the United States and was concerned with medical responses to persons suspected of being dead on arrival. One finding was that patients deemed to be responsible for their condition, for example alcoholics or drug abusers, received less sympathy and less effort was made to revive them than was the case with those who were deemed to be totally 'blameless', e.g. patients with heart-attacks. A British study of patients brought to an accident and emergency department after taking an overdose of drugs, likewise found that ambulance drivers, doctors and nurses, were less sympathetic to them (saying, for example, 'she did it herself') than they were to those brought in with involuntary conditions (Ghodse, 1978).

The attribution of responsibility and blame by lay and professional groups has been investigated by many researchers; less attention has been given to the question of self-blame, that accorded by sick persons to themselves. This issue is of importance for women; feelings of guilt and blame are integral parts of women's lives in contemporary society; responsibility for the health of the family and for the happiness of everyone in it rests on women, and if sickness arises in herself or in one of the others, the woman is likely to regard herself as culpable.

The guilt feelings experienced by women are complex, and are characteristic of women's lives in general, irrespective of illness. Many housewives and mothers are unhappy and dissatisfied with their lives and experience much guilt as a consequence. As women imbibe feminine social roles in childhood, they learn that family life and motherhood are not only the natural goals of women, but their chief source of happiness; it follows that if, with the goal attained, they feel discontented and unfulfilled, the fault is in themselves, and guilt results (Sharpe, 1984). Such feelings are accentuated when husbands, relatives and friends appear to think (as they frequently do) that the woman should be satisfied, and are exacerbated by advertising with its constant theme of the happy housewife and mother smiling, and enjoying her domestic tasks (Millum, 1975). Feeling guilty and aware of social disapproval, most women are naturally reluctant to talk openly about their dissatisfaction with traditional role expectations, thus making the strain worse (Cooperstock and Lennard, 1979).

Not surprisingly, when housewives become depressed, or develop problems which doctors call 'phobias', 'obsessions' or 'anxieties', they feel increasingly guilty and responsible for their condition.

One respondent in Jocelyn Cornwell's study (Cornwell, 1984, p. 151)

> reported that she suffered from anxiety and depression on and off throughout her adult life, and blamed herself for this. She saw the cause of her trouble with 'her nerves' as something inside herself which it was up to her to do something about. When the trouble began, she had been referred to a psychiatrist and at various times since then she had consulted her GP who prescribed tranquillizers... Essentially, she said, her depression could be avoided, provided she was firm with herself and developed the strength of mind and the determination to overcome her own anxieties.

Women interviewed elsewhere frequently took the view that they could not be 'normal' if, having comfortable homes, they were 'nervy' or depressed, and that it must be unnatural for mothers not to be happy and contented with their children (Miles, 1988, p. 64).

Bearing a burden of guilt, women do not feel entitled fully to withdraw from duties and claim the sick role; rather than 'give in', they persevere with the daily routine which, all too often, is at the root of their problems.

Returning to health and duration of the sick role

The duration of withdrawal from social activities on account of sickness is rather a vexed question: it is a matter of negotiation (not always spelt out) between patient, doctor and social group, and is especially ambiguous in cases which do not necessitate hospital admission. Often there is no precise medical advice as to the patient's resumption of activities.

David Mechanic argued that behaviour during an illness episode, and the timing of a return to health, are functions of role obligations (Mechanic, 1982, p. 32):

> whether people go to work, stay in bed, or assume the sick role in some other way, depends not only on their symptoms but also on attitudes toward their obligations and the requirements of their social situation.

Relinquishing the sick role, no less than the original claim to it, is subject to a range of personal, medical and social considerations. Staying in bed is a clear indication of withdrawal from all activities. In studies of differences in sickness behaviour as between men and women, Marcus and her colleagues noted distinct patterns among people who had taken to their beds with sickness during the study period. Women with young children reported lower rates of withdrawal from obligations than did women without children. However, in a sample where only a minority of women had young children, the women maintained the sick role longer than did the men (women averaged 11.82 bed-days, compared to 6.64 for the men). The authors explained these findings by referring to the 'fixed-role hypothesis', i.e. people with more fixed, less flexible, role obligations are likely to maintain the sick role for shorter periods of time than those with less fixed, more flexible role obligations (Marcus and Seeman, 1981; Marcus et al., 1983).

People for whom dependency is distasteful are anxious for a quick return to health. To remain in bed and to rely on others for essential requirements, places an adult in the position of a child; an uncomfortable experience for many, perhaps. A duality of attitudes to dependency was recorded by Jocelyn Cornwell (Cornwell, 1984, p. 139) who found that the working-class men in her study continued to go to work as long as they were able to do so, but at home

> they had no qualms about expecting their wives to be sympathetic whilst they 'gave in' to even fairly mild symptoms. They also seemed to have very little trouble in taking to their beds when they were at home so as to be fit for another day of 'working it off' at work.

These men accepted the need to work, but also enjoyed being looked after on a part-time sick role basis, at home in the evenings. For wives, such indulgence is seldom a possibility: to occupy a sustained part-time sick role in the evenings would be unthinkable for most wives and mothers.

How long to stay in bed, and when to return to normal obligations, can be problematic for women when their symptoms are connected with their reproductive functions. Bed rest and withdrawal from work is a possible response to menstrual pain. Although the World Health Organization survey found that only a minority of women allowed such pain to disrupt their functioning, those who find it necessary to withdraw from work must negotiate the period of that withdrawal, in the sense that the social group will 'understand' that a few days is appropriate in such cases. A recent study of schoolgirls in Finland showed that half of those who experienced severe menstrual pain stayed at home (Teperi and Rimpela, 1989). No doubt the severity of pain, as well as the girls' attitude to school, would play a part here, but negotiations with parents and teachers would have determined the duration of the sick role.

During pregnancy, the usual situation does not apply: it is not only the timing of the return to health but the timing of the original withdrawal from activities that determine the duration of sick role. Doctors currently favour the adoption of a modified sick role, advocating the avoidance of strenuous work, and the giving up of duties, in the latter stages of pregnancy. When to give up work is negotiable, but doctors can be quite decisive (Graham and Oakley, 1986, p. 103):

Patient: I am a hairdresser. I only do three days a week – is it all right to go on working?

Doctor: Up to twenty-eight weeks is all right on the whole, especially if you have a trouble-free pregnancy as you obviously have. After that it's better to give up.

Patient: I only work three days a week, I feel fine.

Doctor: Yes, everything is fine, but now you've got to this stage, it's better to give up, just in case.

Whether to regard withdrawal from work during late pregnancy as the assumption of the sick role is as ambiguous as the consideration of pregnancy as health or sickness, as has been discussed before. When usual activities have to be abandoned, the role certainly resembles the role of the sick. It is arguable that in current Western societies, medicalized pregnancy, like medicalized old age, is easily viewed as a form of 'sickness' for which the sick role is appropriate.

Withdrawal from usual activities during pregnancy, and the timing of that withdrawal, are influenced not only by medical advice but also by social embarrassments and uncomfortable experiences. During a seminar on experiences in pregnancy, one woman said that she gave up teaching when schoolchildren made 'ribald' comments on her shape, and another that she was asked by the head teacher to give up when pupils asked difficult and embarrassing questions. Other women related that their 'bulge' forced them to give up working as barmaids, as entertainers, or as receptionists, all jobs where to be smart, slim and attractive, is a job requirement.

4

Living with long-term health-related problems

Coping with chronic illness and disability

Problems surrounding the processes of assuming, according and learning the sick role in acute illness episodes have been discussed in Chapter 3. In spite of areas of uncertainty and disagreement, occupying the sick role in these instances is frequently uncontroversial in that the sick person is evidently unable to function normally and consequently has to withdraw from work or other responsibilities. Sufferers from pneumonia, influenza or the after-effects of surgery are demonstrably and undeniably 'sick' besides which there is the legitimate expectation that their condition is but temporary. The patient's social group can operate on the assumption that acute sickness is amenable to treatment and that a return to health and to pre-illness social roles can be anticipated. The situation with regard to chronic sickness and disablement is quite else.

The most troublesome of the non-life-threatening problems of ill health today are the long-term conditions – some stable, some episodic, some progressive – congenital or pursuant to illness or injury. Not all of these conditions can be classified as problems to the same extent: medication keeps some of them under control, surgical appliances of advanced design are available, enabling sufferers to lead 'normal' lives. But it is usually a matter of degree and for many, recovery is problematic or out of the question and prospects of improvement in social functioning likewise doubtful or non-existent. Even where there are such expectations, the time-scale is likely to be lengthy.

When individuals and their families accept the presence of multiple sclerosis or arthritis, to name but two examples, or the fact of amputation or paralysis following, say, a car accident or a stroke, they face a long-term, damaging alteration to their life-style. Persons with psychiatric illness and their families suffer this consequence to a marked extent and have in addition to cope with stigma. As with other conditions, psychiatric illnesses can be of varying intensity but they are often of long duration, incapacitating and charged with uncertainty: how long depression or agoraphobia may last, how incapacitating schizophrenia may become, cannot with assurance be predicted.

It is the case, then, that unlike acute illness, a chronic condition has frequently to be reckoned not in terms of a few weeks but of years or even a lifetime, with the consequence that it gives rise to a different set of social expectations. It may not be necessary to desist from all of the activities which the social group would expect of a well member; it is often enough to perform a modified social role, declining or withdrawing from some commitments while fulfilling others. Thus, social expectations as to the behaviour of the sick person cannot be the same in acute and chronic illness: the expectation of a socially legitimated temporary withdrawal from activities is inappropriate as is anticipation of a return to full health. Someone confined to a wheelchair, for example, cannot be expected to act like the able-bodied and the social group will settle for a best possible performance in the circumstances. As with espisodes of acute illness, however, acceptance by the social group that the condition is genuine (or 'legitimate') is essential for maintenance of social relations and for sympathy and assistance to be given to the long-term sick. Freidson (1975a, p. 235) argued that acceptance by the group is conditional on withdrawal from activities and obligations being limited to the minimum necessary for the given condition.

> A chronically ill or permanently impaired person who 'expects too much' or 'makes too many demands' is likely to be rejected by others. In that case, legitimacy is not conditional on seeking help as it is for illness believed to be acute and curable. Rather, legitimacy is conditional on limiting demands for privileges to what others consider appropriate (to what others believe one cannot be held responsible for).

The level to which demands should be kept and the amount of relief necessary to the condition, can be very contentious issues and need constantly to be negotiated in concrete situations between the sick or disabled person and the social group. Thus, the essence of the social experience of chronic illness is ambiguity.

In cases of episodic illness, psychiatric disorder and diseases which

develop slowly and are not always apparent, it is the legitimacy of the
condition itself that may, from time to time, need to be re-affirmed.

With illnesses such as multiple sclerosis, periods of being symptom-
free (or remissions), may alternate with periods of being very ill, and it
can be difficult for friends and relatives to believe that the disease is
always there; legitimacy is constantly undermined by doubts during
symptom-free times (Robinson, 1988, p. 58):

> Some people can't understand why I'm in a wheelchair some-
> times and not other times... with some, as long as I look cheerful
> and say I am feeling fine they can cope with me, but if I say I
> don't feel well they ignore the remark, or say I look well! I feel
> that some of them think I'm being lazy or giving up if I'm in a
> wheelchair...

Illnesses which develop slowly can likewise be the subject of doubts
and uncertainties. The borderline between being well enough to work
and ill enough not to is ill-defined and shifting: if arthritis, for example,
has worsened only slightly, why give up domestic work at this particular time? (Bury, 1988).

Likewise, credibility can be called into question if a condition is not
visible and accounts of pain or distress have to be elicited before they
can be verified and accepted. This is often so in cases of psychiatric
illness: how is the social group of a depressed woman to judge the
extent of her incapacity when the severity of the condition fluctuates
and nothing much can be seen?

Gender has considerable influence on the experience of chronic illness. Because women live longer, there are more women among the
chronic sick elderly, and women are more likely to be living alone
when chronic illness sets in. At all ages, in the negotiations for acceptance, assistance and support, chronic sick women are in a different
position from men. The impact on family life of incapacity in wife or
mother is often dramatic; it is the woman who 'holds the home
together'. The reaction of husband and relatives may well reflect the
essential role of the woman in the family and the difficulty of managing without her. The experience of stigma and rejection differs according to gender; and the employment problems of disabled women and
disabled men are dissimilar.

Problems of legitimacy and credibility loom larger in the illness
experience of women than in that of men. The widely-held stereotyped
picture of woman as complaining, weak and inclined to magnify problems leads to general scepticism about the extent and severity of
women's symptoms. Much less are the symptoms of men called into
question (Nathanson, 1975). Thus, women sufferers from debilitating
conditions such as psychiatric illness, multiple sclerosis or arthritis are

under more pressure than men in similar circumstances to limit their demands on their social group. Often, the sick woman will find herself being exhorted by her husband and relations to 'fight', 'not give in', or 'pull herself together' and 'be brave' (Miles, 1988; Robinson, 1988). Such pressure reflects the group's doubts concerning legitimacy of women's conditions and its expectation that women 'magnify' and 'exaggerate' their problems.

Feelings of guilt, of responsibility in some way for being ill, are more typical of women than of men. Like those with acute illness, the chronic sick try to make sense of their experiences by asking the question 'Why me?' People attempt to think of ways in which the disease could have been avoided. In cases where the cause of the disease is unknown, or where medical practitioners suggest the possibility of psychological factors in causation, feelings of responsibility and blame are accentuated. Research also suggests gender differences in imputations of guilt and blame: husbands of female multiple sclerosis sufferers are more likely to believe that their wives could have avoided the disease than are wives to believe that of their husbands in a similar situation (although it is fair to say that only a minority of both sexes regard multiple sclerosis as avoidable). Husbands of women with psychiatric illness tend at attach blame to their wives while wives of men with a similar condition do not (Miles, 1988; Robinson, 1988).

Feeling guilty for the impact of one's illness on the children is also experienced more by women. Both mothers and fathers typically feel distressed by the negative effects their disability or sickness has on their children ('I am not a real parent'; 'I can't look after them'); but mothers are more likely to blame themselves and feel guilty while fathers tend to be angry and blame 'fate' and external factors for the continuing harm done (Miles, 1978).

Employment problems

Restriction of opportunity in a variety of fields invariably accompanies chronic sickness and disablement and is compounded when stigma attaches to the condition. Peoplr suffering from one or other of these problems face disadvantages in employment, social life, housing, leisure and a wide range of other activities. Of course, it is possible to triumph over adversity and history affords many examples. Franklin Roosevelt, four times elected American President, was paralysed following poliomyelitis, Beethoven was deaf, Van Gogh suffered mental illness, Helen Keller, one of the most remarkable of women, was both blind and deaf yet lived a life of exemplary achievement. It remains true, nevertheless, that most afflicted people have to struggle harder to achieve less, independence is denied them and their status, low.

To maintain oneself is a social imperative and it is in the field of employment that some of the worst difficulties are encountered. Congenitally sick and disabled people know the problems from birth: for previously well individuals their impact is shattering. Disability following injury is likely to hit suddenly and imply immediate job loss; with many other long-term conditions the process is more drawn-out but just as certain. The work may become too strenuous for one with reduced strength or stamina, precision tasks progressively more difficult for someone with arthritis in the hands. A person may be too weak and tired to work full-time (e.g. kidney patients on dialysis; see Morgan, 1988), or incapacitated by psychiatric illness (Wansbrough and Cooper, 1980) or develop functional disabilities (e.g. multiple sclerosis; see Burnfield, 1985). Men who lose their employment in these and similar circumstances will, where practicable, seek alternative, less-demanding, or part-time, jobs; women, on the other hand, are much more likely not to do so but to become 'housewives'.

The employment problems of disabled and chronic sick women present a complex picture, an important element of which is the availability of the 'housewife role' for women who do not engage in paid employment. According to Mildred Blaxter's study (Blaxter, 1976, p. 157), disabled men express more uneasiness about not working than do disabled women, who

> could more easily find other roles which were accepted by their family, their social group and (implicitly, if not formally) by officials as legitimate – doing the housework for parents, or for working daughters, or simply concentrating on their own housekeeping. These might not be the roles that they themselves would choose, of course, and several women expressed almost desperate unhappiness about being unable to keep their jobs, but this distress was based solely on their personal feelings and was never compounded by any pressures from their families, doctors or officials.

There are a number of drawbacks in the availability of the housewife role for women who, without disability, would work in paid employment. Firstly, there is the unhappiness of being an unwilling housewife: Blaxter quotes a woman suffering from myocardial ischaemia, the mother of school-age children (Blaxter, 1976, p. 157):

> The doctor said why don't I stay at home for a bit? I told the doctor last week how bored I was getting – I can't stand being alone all day and maybe I'll start work again. The doctor agreed it's bad for me, getting fussed and not knowing what to do with myself – it'll be grand to get out of the house and have the company.

Another serious disadvantage is that unemployed women are less socially visible than unemployed men, with the result that their rehabilitation and long-term future are given less consideration. Because women have an alternative role, it can easily be accepted that their staying at home and not having paid employment is the norm so that they tend to get less help from health professionals and less encouragement from families, officials and employers to overcome handicaps and return to work. Lack of active rehabilitation programmes can lead to hopeless unemployment.

The structure of women's employment has a bearing on the job experiences of disabled women. Many, especially mothers of pre-school and school-age children, look for 'convenient' jobs, which will fit in with domestic duties, a shorter day and a close-to-home location taking precedence over rates of pay, prospects and job-satisfaction. The service sector (catering, laundry, cleaning, small shops), domestic work, and small offices, where labour turnover is high, offer to women a range of jobs which can be done part-time or at odd hours. Such employers are to be found in most areas and are often more flexible than 'big firms' over such matters as school holidays and children's sickness, but the rates of pay are typically low (Sharpe, 1984). In such settings, special arrangements can be made when women employees develop chronic sickness or disability: flexible working hours and convenient working conditions can be negotiated within a personal and sympathetic relationship, e.g. Beryl, 33 years old, a chronic agoraphobic (Miles, 1988, p. 60):

> I've worked for the same family for the last two years. I go there twice a week, it's easy because no one is at home, they are all out at business. I also put my name down at the school to do school meals but had to wait for years, there is always a waiting list. The school is just round the corner, and the family live in the street next to it. I couldn't travel in a bus, it has to be local work for me.

The case of Frances, 40 years old, with depression lasting for several years is reported by Miles also (1988, p. 61):

> It is a small shop, open very long hours and the owner is very good. When I had to go to group therapy in the afternoons, we agreed that I would make it up on Sunday mornings. One week I couldn't work at all, but the week after I went in early mornings as well. Not every employer would agree to that.

The case of Mrs. Macandrew, who worked in a department store and was injured in a road accident is reported by Blaxter (1976, p. 158):

The manager suggested that I stay off work until after the summer, my job'll always be waiting, and that would be most convenient for them, and I'm not in a particular hurry.

Typically, people suffering from disabilities or chronic sickness experience downward mobility in employment, having to accept lesser jobs than the ones they held previously. Beryl (above) was a trained and experienced secretary but, with twin children at home and an agoraphobic aversion to public transport, her choices were restricted and she had little option but to take up domestic work. Limited opportunities, low pay and no prospects characterize the employment situation of these people with the women, if anything, being even worse off than the men.

Restriction of employment possibilities is not always attributable to the chronic condition as such, it derives also from low self-esteem and loss of confidence pursuant to it. Those with visible conditions, or psychiatric illness, are conscious of stigma which they tend to anticipate and often experience. Even without this extra burden, people who have not worked outside of their homes for a lengthy period, especially if due to illness or injury, are inclined to doubt their ability to find work again. Such difficulties confront both sexes but they are additional to the disadvantages at the workplace which even healthy and able-bodied women have to contend with as they struggle to overcome the male stereotype of them as weaker and less employable than men.

It is interesting to observe that with regard to paid employment, single women often experience treatment by the social group which resembles that accorded to married women rather than to employable men. Families and health professionals alike are apt to assume that they can stay at home, without bothering about employment while developing a long-term sickness. Being in the home, perhaps with parents or adult daughters, is viewed as a proper and acceptable role for single women. Advice to 'stay at home' would rarely be given to a man under retirement age unless the impairment was severe; it is often given to women with quite mild forms of sickness (Roberts, 1985).

Seeking and receiving social support

The meaning of social support

Long-term illness and disability increase demands on the immediate social groups of both women and men. The nature of an individual's social circle has a bearing on the extent to which demands can be made and be found acceptable: the social circle may range from extensive to narrow and relationships within it may be deep and permanent or shallow and transitory.

When present-day researchers study the social relationships of long-term sick and disabled people, they build on the findings of social scientists, who, since the mid-twentieth century have directed their attention to individuals' relationships with members of their social circle and to the connection between the strength of such social ties, or want of them, and personal health. Some of these studies will be considered before turning to the social relationships of chronic sick and disabled women.

A conceptual tool, the 'social network' was developed in an early study by Elizabeth Bott (1957) and has been much used by later researchers. Bott argued that in contemporary industrial societies, the typical small family is connected with a number of individuals and groups (which may be, but are not necessarily, connected with each other) which, together form a network. This network has an 'informal' component, made up of relatives, friends, colleagues and neighbours, and a 'formal' component comprising voluntary associations, professionals (e.g. doctor, teacher, priest), and other contacts. Models and measures of social networks have been developed and characteristics such as diversity, reciprocity, density and interrelatedness (i.e. the extent to which the members of a person's informal network also know each other), have been described.

The support, assistance, and affection, received and given, are considered to play an important part in an individual's life: evidence suggests that social support can act as a buffer against stress, cushioning its impact (Dean and Lin, 1977; Bloom, 1982) and that social support has a direct, positive effect on psychological well-being (Klerman, 1978; Henderson *et al.*, 1980; Mueller, 1980). Longitudinal studies have pointed to an association between social support and mortality: the Alameda County Study reported that in a nine-year follow-up period, people who had strong social and community ties were less likely to die prematurely than those with lesser contacts (Berkman and Syme, 1979); this finding was confirmed by the 'Tecumsch ' study which also showed that an association between strong social support and reduced mortality rates applies to people of diverse occupational groups and age groups, and cuts across overall health status (House *et al.*, 1982). Social support may also influence the progression of diseases, and there is evidence to show that good social support can improve adjustment, lessen the risk of complications and increase the chances of recovery (Vaughn and Leff, 1976; Venters, 1981; Funch and Mettlin, 1982).

What constitutes good social support? The difficulty is that the notion lacks conceptual clarity and is difficult to assess in research.

Everyone enters into social relationships because people live in society and not in isolation, but the notion of social support suggests more than being a member of society and depending somewhat nebulously on other members of it. Perhaps the best approach to understanding social support is to regard it as having both an emotional (or 'affective') and a practical (or 'instrumental') content, the one representing the provision of affection and sympathy, creating in its object a sense of belonging, of being loved and needed, the other, the provision of assistance, financial, physical or material. Both emotional and practical support can be strong or weak in terms of quality and quantity, and it is important to make a distinction. Quantitative support may come from one or many network members, and vary from slight to substantial. Support may also vary qualitatively: emotional ties can be intense or shallow and practical assistance may be given cheerfully and willingly or with reluctance. Thus, the nature of the social support that an individual receives will always differ in some degree from that received by another (Pilisuk and Froland, 1978).

Research into social support and health is beginning to distinguish between the components of support and their separate effects on the aetiology and course of diseases. Thus, Brown and his colleagues have consistently shown that one kind of emotional support, that provided by an intimate confidante, plays an important part in preventing depression (Brown *et al.*, 1986) and Thoits suggested that emotional support has greater predictive power than practical support in psychological disorders (Thoits, 1983).

Methodological problems and the diversity of measures and conceptual tools used by researchers make overall evaluation of studies difficult. A variety of definitions of social support have been used in various studies: some researchers were interested in integration within a community, others in the quality and strength of social ties and others again in the actual support provided. In some studies individuals' perceptions of the support they received and their satisfaction with it were explored; in others, some objective measures were attempted, such as frequency of contact or information from both providers and recipients of support. Some researchers developed complex quantified scales and measures of attachments. However, from these diverse studies a clear message would seem to emerge: maintaining social ties and receiving support are conducive to good health as well as being vitally important for those suffering from illness.

Gender differences in both giving and obtaining support are marked, and the association between social ties, support, and health also varies according to gender. On the latter point, there is evidence to show that the relationship between lack of social support and both psychological and somatic distress is stronger for women than for men (Henderson,

1974); in the Alameda Study it was found that lack of support, and isolation, were associated with increased mortality for women (Berkman and Syme, 1979); other researchers on specific samples suggested that an association between social support and well-being is more marked for females. Likewise, in the recent British *Health and Life-style Survey*, where 'perceived' social support was studied (on the grounds that it was found in previous research to be most consistently related to health) the results showed a clear association between levels of this kind of support and reported 'malaise'. A high proportion (60 per cent) of women with severe lack of support reported a high rate of malaise; the findings pointed the same way for men, but to a lesser degree (Stark, 1987). Thus it seems likely that although social ties and support are important to women and men, they mean more to women, whose health correspondingly is more affected by a lack thereof.

Women are the most likely providers of support: this is the conclusion of investigations covering a wide field. Studies of primate behaviour, human evolution, developmental studies, and parenting behaviour, all suggest that women are more skilled, more able, and more interested in giving support to others, both children and adults. (For a review of the literature, see Flaherty and Richman, 1989.) This conclusion is confirmed by studies of carers: in contemporary western societies, it is the women who provide care and support (Graham, 1983; Ungerson, 1987).

Less researched is the important question of obtaining support: how do women obtain help in sickness?; how much support do they receive?; and whom do they turn to when in need?

Emotional support

Emotional (or affective) support is of considerable importance to those people experiencing long-term illness, either physical or mental, although in the past it was researchers exploring the implications of mental illness who paid more attention to it. Only in recent years has emotional support for people with chronic physical conditions been increasingly investigated.

Women, who form the majority of those endeavouring to cope with depression, agoraphobia, and chronic anxiety states, paint a bleak picture when asked to describe the level of emotional support that they are getting. Susannah Ginsberg and George Brown (1982) looked at the support accorded by family and friends to severely depressed women (who were encouraged to talk about themselves) and their findings were, indeed, bleak. Three-quarters of the women felt that they received little or no support from mothers, other relatives, or friends;

three-quarters of the women who lived with their husbands likewise reported minimal support or none at all. Another study (Miles, 1988) came up with similar results: women with neurotic problems (depression, agoraphobia, etc.) reported weak and unsatisfactory emotional support.

Do these women try to obtain support? Do they try to discuss their problems with members of their own personal social network? The answer is that they do: women, more than men, with long-term problems, feel the need to confide in others; unfortunately they seldom find the support they are seeking.

Whom do people turn to for emotional support? In a study by Horwitz in the United States, based on interviews with 120 patients at a community mental health centre in New Haven, women and men were asked to give information concerning the members of their network with whom they had discussed the problems which brought them to psychiatric treatment. In another study, by Miles (1988), also based on interviews with 85 people treated for psychiatric illness, respondents were asked to whom they turned for emotional support, whom they could confide in and talk to. According to these studies spouses are frequently chosen as a first resort, partly because their physical proximity makes the approach easy and practicable and partly because cultural expectations in contemporary society decree that spouses share in each other's concerns. Most researchers find, however, that wives are more often mentioned than husbands as confidantes and that husbands, although approached, seldom prove to be the primary source of support for their wives (see also Vernoff *et al.*, 1981; Kessler, 1985). In Miles's study it was found that the majority of the women made efforts to gain the support of their husbands in time of need, e.g. when they felt especially low, or experienced panic attacks, or when decisions had to be made, but they mostly reported failure. Likewise, in the study of Ginsberg and Brown, women suffering from depression, who lived with their husbands, were generally unsuccessful in gaining support. They said of their husbands, 'He doesn't want to know', 'He doesn't want to hear' or 'It goes in one ear and out the other' (Ginsberg and Brown, 1982, p. 95); other women confirm these experiences:

> There is only my husband. I wish there was someone else. Mostly, I keep my thoughts to myself. I hoard my thoughts, then I get upset and tell my husband, because there is nobody else. I usually regret it afterwards.

According to Miles (1988, p. 95):

> My husband is there but he doesn't want to talk. He doesn't understand. He just says 'don't bother me'.

Thus, the quality of support available is often weak.

By contrast, men who turn to their wives receive a more satisfactory level of emotional support. This is not surprising; indeed, it is part of cultural expectations that women provide love, tenderness and interest and, as discussed previously, are the more skilful providers of affective support.

It is also possible that the failure of many husbands to appreciate their wives' need for support and their unwillingness to discuss with them issues of feelings and emotions, are rooted in Western cultural norms. Men would not discuss such matters with each other in clubs and pubs – that would be 'women's talk'. Expressions of care, tenderness and affection can be regarded as 'unmanly'. Such cultural norms of behaviour result in men obtaining emotional support from their wives but not from male friends and relatives, and women tending to receive emotional support not from their husbands, but from female friends and relations.

It needs to be borne in mind that lack of support is a contributory factor in the onset of mental illness. Indeed, it is axiomatic that the happily married are less likely to become depressed than are those whose marriages have gone stale (Brown and Harris, 1978). Even so, confirmation of wives' lack of success in obtaining emotional support from their husbands, in cases of illness, derives from many studies exploring, not only long-term conditions but shorter-term illnesses and post-operative recovery. For example, Christine Webb studied social support for women who had undergone hysterectomy (Webb and Wilson-Barnett, 1983; Webb, 1986); she asked women how their partners felt about their having the operation and found that more than half of those living with a male partner simply did not know his opinion of the operation. Those who did know what the men thought reported positive and negative views in equal proportion. One woman's reply was representative of many: 'I don't know. He has never actually said. I don't think he was bothered really.' (Webb, 1986, p. 102.)

Other than spouses, relatives and friends may be approached in the hope of obtaining emotional support. Horvitz's research showed that women are more active than men in trying to utilize members of their network for talks about their problems, a finding borne out by other studies (Miller and Ingham, 1976; Hirsch, 1979; Stone and Neal, 1984). This is interesting because those women who lack employment beyond the confines of their homes thereby tend to have smaller social networks than do men whose workmates form part of their networks. But men, as we have seen, are more likely than women to obtain solace from their spouses.

Another feature of support seeking from friends and relatives is that usually a person of the same sex is chosen. Women frequently find that emotional support from female friends and kin is more easily obtained and is qualitatively better than that obtained from husbands. Women are more interested in exchanging confidences, thus (Webb, 1986, p. 102):

> I think Margaret has been the most helpful because she sits down and has a chat. Not just about the operation, you know, like she sits and has a chat about everything. You need somebody to talk to and she has been great.

In an interview study of elderly people's supportive networks, carried out in Wales by Clare Wenger (1984), the respondents were asked whom they would turn to if they felt 'down' and wanted to talk to someone. The women relied more on friends and neighbours than did the men, irrespective of marital status. Perhaps the most interesting result was that it was the elderly married women who relied most heavily (45 per cent) on friends and neighbours for talks. It seems that in old age, too, emotional support for women is more likely to come from other women than from men.

However, this does not mean that all women actually find this kind of support; on the contrary, as mentioned before, Ginsberg and Brown (1982) noted three-quarters of the depressed women in their sample feeling that they received little or no support from relatives and friends, and other research also paints a bleak picture. In Webb's 1986 study of hysterectomy patients, 20 out of 50 women had no confidante of any kind with whom they could talk over their worries, and some, not even a 'sympathetic' family.

There are a number of barriers to successfully gaining emotional support. One is the perceived need by women help-seekers to protect their near relations (mothers, sisters and grown-up daughters) from distress; this prevents them from seeking support from these sources.

Ginsberg and Brown found that only half of the depressed women in their sample attempted to talk about their depression to their mothers. The reason usually given is the wish not to upset mother. Comments such as 'I don't want to worry her' and 'I don't want to burden her, she's got enough worries' are frequently made. The perceived need to protect near family from burdens and anxieties also serves to restrict the imparting of confidences to adult daughters and to sisters.

There are other barriers to obtaining emotional support: women with psychiatric problems try to look for others who not are only willing to provide affection but understand the nature of, for example, depression or agoraphobia. This is not easy (Ginsberg and Brown, 1982, p. 96):

I have talked to one friend a bit about the way I felt . . . but she really had no concept of the extent of my depression or the extent of my inability to cope or my feelings of inadequacy. Perhaps this is a problem – how do you explain it to people who've never felt this way? How do you tell someone the size of the Empire State Building if they've never seen a tall building?

And Miles (1988, p. 98):

No one can understand agoraphobia who hasn't experienced it. My Mum tried and my brothers tried but they can't and I can't explain to them . . . even if you do experience it you can't really understand somebody else, it's different for different people.

Nevertheless, most support-seekers find that people with personal experience of their particular type of problem come nearest to understanding and are the best choice for emotional support, provided, of course, such are available. The more common is the problem, the more likely it is that a fellow sufferer within the social network can be located. But serious mental illness is completely outside the experience of most people who consequently lack the capacity to empathize.

Those suffering from long-term physical conditions also experience difficulty in finding potential providers of support who can understand the feelings of someone suffering from a particular disease or disability. To try to explain the experience of multiple sclerosis or arthritis can also be likened to attempts to describe the Empire State Building to a desert dweller. Indeed, Robinson found that only 14 per cent of women multiple sclerosis sufferers thought that others could understand the situation of persons with the disease 'very well' or 'quite well' (Robinson, 1988), and it is interesting to note that women were more pessimistic about the capacity of others to understand than were the men, of whom 32 per cent answered positively.

Chronic sick and disabled people (like other minority groups in society) have the possibility to seek the company of those in a similar situation to themselves. There exist in most Western countries, clubs and societies with branches in many localities, where it is possible for those afflicted to meet others in like case. In the early 1960s, Erving Goffman described many such organisations which had, among their aims, the provision of understanding and support (Goffman, 1963, p. 22):

. . . then there are the huddle-together self-help clubs, formed by the divorced, the aged, the obese, the physically handicapped, the iliostomied and colostomied. There are residential clubs, voluntary to varying degrees, formed for the ex-alcoholic and ex-addict. There are national associations such as the AA . . .

The notion of self-help has since become even more popular, and many associations for people with a single disease have been formed, e.g. the Multiple Sclerosis Society and the Parkinson's Disease Society. The main objective of self-help groups and associations may be practical assistance, information exchange, or treatment. But even where emotional support is not the main objective, it may well be a by-product of the gathering: the feeling that one is not alone, that others can understand what one is going through, relieves the sense of isolation. There is a chance of meeting someone with whom friendship and mutual support can be established.

For a chronic-sick person to be in a position to find the companionship of fellow sufferers, first the diagnosis has to be confirmed, then the relevant association/group/society has to be located, and lastly, means of getting to and from meeting places need to be found, success depending on the willingness of others around them to provide assistance. In this context it is unhelpful to women that doctors are more reluctant to reveal their diagnosis to them than they are to their male patients. However, women are more likely than men to discover the diagnosis for themselves, as indicated by the findings of studies of multiple sclerosis (Robinson, 1988; Miles, 1978): doctors are more inclined to engage in the stratagem of 'managed discovery' with their female patients, i.e. try to manoeuvre the discovery by the patient at some chosen 'propitious' time (Brunel ARMS Research Unit, 1983).

Women, possibly because of greater difficulties in getting a firm diagnosis, are more likely to feel relief when they are told what it is they suffer from: Robinson found that a higher proportion of women than men experienced relief when the diagnosis of multiple sclerosis was established (Robinson, 1988). That anyone should be relieved by such a diagnosis may seem paradoxical, but at least discovery of the diagnosis paves the way towards the finding of fellow sufferers. Women with 'mystery-symptoms' especially, experience a sense of relief when a name is given to their condition and they can set about finding others with similar problems: for example, for agoraphobic women, the realization that there are others with similar experiences of panic and anxiety is a first step in reducing loneliness and getting support (Brown, 1986).

Support from fellow sufferers is important for another reason in that it constitutes a way of utilizing the relevant experience of the social group and of obtaining indications as to the 'right', socially approved, ways of acting in a particular sick role situation. In struggling to understand and attach meaning to suffering, in trying to decide whether to continue with treatment, or whether fighting or accepting the disease is more appropriate and approved, sufferers have recourse to the meanings, explanations and actions provided by their group culture, and obtainable through discussions with fellow sufferers (Miles, 1988, p. 100):

> I didn't know what to do, will people think I am giving in if I start group therapy? Is it better to fight it alone? Then I found a friend in Tracy, she even lived near me, and she encouraged me to go to group-sessions.

> It was a comfort to know someone who had experienced it. I was desperately upset at first, I thought nobody can be in such a state who is not mad...I thought I was going mad, I was frightened. It was such a relief to tell all about it to Meg, she had panic attacks herself. She went to a psychologist and he really helped her, so I thought I am doing the right thing...when I get too panicky now I ring Meg and she says 'I know how you are feeling'. It's odd what a difference it makes.

People vary in their wish to confide in others and in their evaluations of the quantity and quality of the emotional support they receive. Not only do individuals differ in their assessment of how much support they feel to be adequate, but the cultural valuation placed on the giving and receiving of emotional support also varies. The values of intimacy and 'unburdening' may compete with the values of independence and reserve.

Practical help and assistance

Practical help and assistance (instrumental support) is of the utmost importance in the lives of people disabled by physical or mental illness, injury or deformity; indeed, concerns of obtaining, maintaining and reciprocating assistance dominate the lives of many who find themselves in a dependent situation.

The problems with which people need practical help vary from all personal care in the case of the severely incapacitated to daily help with specific tasks or occasional assistance for those whose functioning is less impaired. In a careful and imaginative British survey of the problems experienced by disabled people, Mildred Blaxter (1976) noted (p. 56) that the 'most remarkable impression is of the great variety of problems of immediate care which arise, and the wide spectrum of sorts of people involved'. Problems can arise in different age groups. The old and sick may be alone and isolated. The young disabled mother may be unable to care for her children. They may vary according to social class – the working-class disabled struggle with lack of economic resources, while mobile professionals may lack supportive kin group and friends living near them. However, according to Mildred Blaxter (1976, p. 57)

> in the sample as a whole, the only personal characteristics that distinguished those whose care presented problems (besides, of course, the severity and nature of their illness or disability) were sex and household composition. Curiously, there were more problems amongst women (51 per cent of all women) than among men (16 per cent of all men). Men would, of course, be more likely to have a non-working spouse at home. Oddly, the definition of 'need' in this respect as used by ward sisters and others in the hospital appeared to assume that women were *less* likely than men to have problems about their after-care: according to the patients' accounts, men were more frequently asked about their arrangements than were women. [original emphasis]

Carers for the sick, the disabled, and the frail elderly, are overwhelmingly female: wives, daughters and sisters provide practical help. How do women obtain their assistance? A considerable problem for many women who need practical help is the minimization of their need by the social group around them. This is especially experienced by young disabled women, who are engaged in full-time domestic work, and are prevented by their condition from caring for children and carrying out domestic tasks. The general assumption made by kin group, health professionals and other network members, is that the needs of those at home are less than are experienced by those at work. Blaxter noted that general practitioners were less sympathetic to young housewives' needs than, for example, those of the elderly, and that few young wives and mothers had the benefit of 'home-help' arrangements. The assumption that the woman in her own home can 'manage' is an aspect of the view, prevalent in society but shown by research to be false, that domestic work is easier to perform than paid employment, that it lends itself with greater facility to flexible work routines, and can be organized to suit the wishes of the housewife (Oakley, 1974).

Another difficulty is the similarly accepted view that disabled people living with their spouses have few practical problems requiring outside assistance; the spouse is available to help. This view may be true of disabled men living with their wives, but not of disabled women whose husbands are usually in full-time employment, and even though willing to provide practical help, are unable to do so. Where young children need care, and the situation in the home becomes desperate, the only way for husbands to attend to necessary domestic tasks is to take time off work, a measure which depends on the nature of their work and may lead to financial problems and even loss of employment. Thus, disabled and chronic sick wives may experience severe problems with their daily practical needs.

This tendency to minimize the needs of such women results in less assistance from professional services and increased reliance on the informal social network. Women whose incapacity to carry out their domestic tasks results from psychiatric problems, fare worst. As discussed previously (Chapter 2), emotional, pyschological, and psychiatric, problems are seen as less 'genuine' and less 'real' than physical conditions, a view shared by officials, friends and relatives alike. A housing official in Mildred Blaxter's study remarked that (Blaxter, 1976, p. 77)

> this 'depression' thing can be overdone. It's amazing how frequently our least-deserving tenants manage to get a diagnosis. We have to be fair to the good tenants, after all.

Such views contribute to lack of assistance. No doubt housing and other welfare agencies have a number of less-than-genuine claims to contend with, but the reality for women with psychiatric problems is that practical help is often badly needed. Agoraphobic mothers need help with taking children to school, with shopping or with routine visits to doctors and dentists for their children and themselves (Brown, 1986). The seriously depressed are likely to need help with caring for young children. Many women need to attend treatment sessions, not necessarily close to home, and can do so only if help with their children is forthcoming.

Where there is much incapacity, practical assistance is provided by husbands, before and after their work, but mostly it comes from female members of the family. Blaxter (1976) noted that, typically, patients underestimated the amount of daily care that they needed, especially while still in hospital and wanting to go home. In her study women, especially, minimized their difficulties and tended to say that 'of course, my daughter/sister/mother will manage' (pp. 58–59). No doubt many reassured themselves thus because they were anxious to be at home, but possibly, too, they lacked personal experience of not being able to 'manage' and shared the accepted view that it is women's duty to help. Once at home, the magnitude of functional incapacity becomes evident, but the assumption that female relatives will help manage, remains.

It is interesting to note that women who have had experience of what it is to cope with disability are much less optimistic than those newly facing it. Also, ability to cope well with multiple sclerosis, for example, is perceived less optimistically by women sufferers than by men; women's perceptions both of the problems they experience and the means of coping with them are more pessimistic than those of men

(Robinson, 1988). This is understandable, as women tend to receive less help and to feel more alone.

The assistance people receive from their social network tends to reflect the domestic division of labour in society, and this is true of the elderly as well as the young. Women receive less help with household tasks which have the stereotype of being 'women's work', such as cooking, ironing, and laundry, whereas women unable to carry out household maintenance or gardening find that assistance is more forthcoming (Wenger, 1984). This pattern, too, may be partly due to minimization of problems, the social group feeling that women's traditional jobs can still be done by a woman, even if disabled, and the woman concerned resisting the notion that she needs help with tasks that she has always performed.

Recipients of help are typically afraid of becoming a burden on their social network. A constant dread of placing too many demands on friends and relations characterizes the social relationships of the long-term sick and disabled. Behind this dread is the insecurity of dependence, the anxiety that by imposing too much on them, help-givers may become resentful and reduce or even withdraw their assistance (Blaxter, 1976, p. 57):

> Mrs Macandrew...seemed to think she had run out of credit, and was reluctant to accumulate too large a 'debt': 'It's gone on far too long now, and I don't want to be beholden: I'll just have to try and manage more myself.'

And Shearer (1981, p. 44)

> One must not show one's feelings of irritation, envy and boredom, in case one loses a useful source of help. No doubt you have noticed that many disabled people are always cheerful, smiling and joking. This is because they know it is the only way to get people to help them.

Also, behind the fear of becoming a burden, and so losing the help provided by others, lies one of the main barriers to seeking the assistance of the social network, namely an inability to reciprocate. Seeking assistance on a reciprocal basis is straightforward: taking turns in accompanying children to school, and baby minding while parents enjoy the odd evening out, are examples. Even help given to someone in acute illness is potentially reciprocal, but the permanently disabled and the progressively sick can never return favours in kind.

Another barrier is the indefinite duration of the need. Even in conditions where cure is possible (and in most cases it is not) the impossibility of estimating the duration of the illness is a problem. Thus, a neighbour who agreed to take the children of an agoraphobic mother to school, would have to continue the service indefinitely. This is why Mrs Macandrew, previously quoted, talked about 'accumulation of debts' and 'running out of credit' (Blaxter, 1976); and a woman suffering from rheumatoid arthritis felt anxiously that she was reaching the 'limits of tolerance' at her home (Bury, 1988). A severely depressed mother said (Miles, 1988, p. 109):

> A lot of people helped after Terry was born and I had post-natal depression. My cousin came down from the North, and others, too ... but when the depression went on, they stopped. People are kind at first but they expect you to recover very quickly, and lose patience. Even my Mum thought I was lazy and a hypochondriac, she said it was time I pulled myself together. You can't ask people to help you all the time, they get tired of you, and don't want to know.

The fear of not being able to reciprocate assistance is not necessarily based on reality. Women with functional incapacity, needing help with many aspects of practical daily life, may reciprocate assistance by offering emotional support, and by willingness to talk to their helpers. Wives who need practical support from husbands, reciprocate by giving affective support. Moreover, sufferers from episodic illness and the frail or chronic-sick elderly, may still help those even more in need of assistance. Again, there are possibilities of mutual support, and a number of examples are given by Clare Wenger: a widow of over 80 who lived alone with her mentally handicapped niece, aged 75, and another widow in her late seventies and not in good health who lived with her daughter, chair-bound, suffering from rheumatoid arthritis (Wenger, 1984, pp. 114–115). Many women who are sick and disabled tend to underestimate their ability to give and devalue what they are able to offer. Women have been brought up to regard their contributions as of lesser value than those of men, often saying, 'I am only a housewife'. It is also the case that practical assistance is frequently valued above emotional support, because it reflects the male domain of activity, rather than the female domain of affections and feelings.

The quantity and quality of support a person can obtain depends a great deal on the kind of social network that is looked to for that support. Geographically-mobile people find difficulty in obtaining daily help from kin and friends, as many of them live at some distance: newcomers to communities, especially dormitory suburbs and similar, find it difficult to establish social ties. Several studies show that length of residence in a locality has a close relationship with the extent of local networks and quantity of support (Walker, 1975); researchers of retirement migration find that loneliness can be a problem for the newly-arrived (Whittington, 1977). Moving to a new locality is quite usual for the physically disabled as adapting an existing home for someone wheelchair-bound (by way of example) can be more difficult than finding a more suitable house elsewhere. This is unfortunate, as a study of multiple sclerosis sufferers suggests that those who continue to live in the same area they had lived in before the illness set in (rural areas especially) receive more help than do newcomers to a district. Long-established residents are known to many people in the area, relatives often live close at hand (Miles, 1979). Immigrants often live in a social world which consists of their fellow immigrants and close ties bind them together; when extensive help and support is needed, the network is able to provide it – this is suggested by studies such as Caroline Currer's on depression and Pathan mothers living in Britain, and Joan Ablon's on a group of Samoan people living in the United States, who suffered severe burns in a fire disaster (Currer, 1986; Ablon, 1986).

Coping with stigma and rejection

The stigma of chronic illness and disability

The term 'stigma' refers to an attribute which is singled out by society and evaluated as undesirable; it devalues the person who possesses it. According to a study by Goffman (1963, p. 2) which has influenced the thinking of social scientists about stigma during the last 25 years,

> society establishes the means of categorising persons and the complement of attributes felt to be ordinary and natural for members of each of these categories. Social settings establish the categories of persons likely to be encountered there. The routines of social intercourse in established settings allow us to deal with anticipated others without special attention or thought.

Goffman goes on to say that on meeting a stranger for the first time, appearances are likely to enable us to anticipate his or her attributes and 'social identity'; in some cases it may become apparent that the stranger possesses an attribute, or trait, which is likely to make others regard that stranger as less than desirable, e.g. as 'tainted, dangerous, weak, or bad'. From being considered whole, usual and ordinary, the person becomes a discounted and devalued one (Goffman, 1962, p. 3):

> Such an attribute is a stigma especially when its discrediting effect is very extensive; sometimes it is also called a failing, a shortcoming, a handicap. It constitutes a special discrepancy between virtual and actual social identity.

Stigma in Goffman's term is an undesirable differentness from what the non-stigmatized have anticipated. The social consequences of being stigmatized are severe: reduced opportunities, discrimination, even outright rejection, typically follow.

There are many kinds of stigma; the concern here is with that attached to physical disability, deformity, disfigurement, chronic illness and mental illness (other kinds of stigma, outside the scope of the present discussion, include those attached to criminals and prostitutes, for example, or to particular ethnic and religious minorities). What matters, in all cases, is society's evaluation of one or other attribute as stigmatizing: stigma is not inherent in any trait or characteristic. Evaluation is specific to place and time; in different societies, at different times, the epileptic, blind, deaf, or mentally handicapped, may or may not be stigmatized.

In a sense, all types of illness are stigmatizing (Hopper, 1981). If stigma is accepted to mean 'undesirable differentness', then any illness comes into this category, with 'serious', long-standing and disabling diseases being more undesirable than slight, short-term and self-limiting conditions. It is helpful to think in terms of a continuum of illnesses: with colds and backaches, for instance, being regarded as part of life, compatible with overall good health (see Chapter 2) and with rheumatoid arthritis, polio and mental illness, outside of the common experience, singling out their victims as unfortunates who are different from other people.

A number of features are common to all types of stigma. The person concerned tends to be defined in terms of the single stigmatizing attribute: for example, a woman of 35, mother of two children, teacher of music, with brown hair and blue eyes, becomes the 'crippled woman'. The stigma tends to override other characteristics and social roles. To possess an attribute which is stigmatized means that the entire person becomes stigmatized. In Goffman's words, the stigma 'spreads' to the whole person and 'spoils' the person's identity.

An important feature of stigma is that it threatens social expectations and the taken-for-granted world of social interaction. People have expectations as to how others will act in given situations and these expectations enable them to orientate their own behaviour towards the anticipated actions of those others. Social expectations are built up slowly and are based on accumulated past experience: routines of daily life and everyday interaction would not be possible without them. For example, a woman entering a grocery shop has a set of expectations, which are taken for granted, not spelt out or verbalized, but nevertheless, strongly held, e.g. that the shopkeeper will be willing to serve her groceries, that money is acceptable in exchange for goods, that the shopkeeper will not be rude, etc. The shopper will feel confident of sharing these expectations with the shopkeeper, even though she may never have entered that particular shop before.

The possession of a differentness, or stigma, signals to others that the possessor is different and that customary expectations should not be assumed. People become unsure of what to expect and this uncertainty disrupts taken-for-granted interactions. If the shopper is uncertain as to how to behave towards a shopkeeper who is restricted to a wheelchair, or what to expect from one who has been in a mental hospital, she may refrain from entering the shop and choose another. Undermined social expectations lead not only to disruption of social interaction, but to rejection.

Why are particular attributes singled out for stigma? The reasons vary. Deformities and disfigurements are highly visible: in a society where good looks, an unblemished physical appearance and wholesomeness are important social values, the opposite extremes are regarded as distasteful, ugly and off-putting. Moreover, beauty is equated with goodness, ugliness with sin. Cinderella is beautiful and virtuous, her sisters are ugly and vicious. Quasimodo is reviled *because* he is a hunchback, yet is capable of love as other men. Loss of limb, paralysis, restricted movement, limping, all signal physical weakness in societies where strength is valued. In the United States and Western Europe, for example, where individual effort and personal achievement are valued, persons suffering from permanent ill-health or other disabilities are less likely to be successful, less likely to achieve socially valued positions and they are regarded as 'less' than the able-bodied and healthy (Parsons, 1951). In achievement-orientated societies dependency acquires stigma: the sick, the disabled and the frail elderly are in a dependent position, like children, and need the help of the healthy, able-bodied adults (Wenger, 1984).

Mental illness traditionally has been much stigmatized in western societies, being evaluated very negatively. Discrimination and rejection is frequently the lot of the psychiatric patient and connotations of unpredictability and inexplicable behaviour accompany mental illness to a greater extent than they do most other stigmatized conditions and are destructive of social expectations. Mental illness (together, perhaps, with severe facial disfigurement) lies at the far end of the continuum of stigmatized conditions. Mildred Blaxter (1976) noted (in her study of the meaning of disability), that feelings of being stigmatized are strongest when the world of everyday interaction is threatened (Blaxter, 1976, p. 198):

> The limited range of 'normal' physical characteristics on which
> the rules of social interaction depend could, it seemed, encom-
> pass to some degree the lack of mobility of those with crippling
> conditions, but any condition which made communication dif-

ficult, or involved unusual or unpredictable behaviour which disrupted the customary pattern of social life, fell too far outside the accepted range...The people in the sample who felt most strongly that their disability was a stigma were those suffering from ataxias, spasticity, severe multiple sclerosis, deafness, blindness to a lesser extent, and epilepsy. It may be conjectured that severe disfigurement, of which there was no example in the sample, ought to be added to the list.

Blaxter found that conditions which were popularly seen as involving 'the brain', 'the nerves' and 'intelligence' were less favourably evaluated than those regarded as physical.

Many people would like to think that the stigma of illness is lessening, but evidence shows otherwise: the form that discrimination takes may be changing, but stigma is still evident. For example, studies concerning mental illness report profound apprehension and rejection of psychiatric patients (Moss and Davidson, 1982; Rahav *et al.*, 1984), a pattern of fear and perceptions of the mentally ill as unpredictable, dangerous and uncanny (Brockman *et al.*, 1979; Leighton, 1984).

Although there has been a considerable amount of research in the field of stigmatized illness, there remain major gaps in current knowledge, among them gender differences in stigmatization and in the consequences of stigma. Serious problems face researchers in designing and carrying out empirical studies in this field. It is difficult to operationalize the concept of stigma and to separate the various elements inherent in the situation of a stigmatized person. An individual's perceptions of being rejected or discriminated against, or regarded as inferior, or unacceptable, because of a stigmatized attribute, is distinguishable from that individual's anxieties and apprehension that such stigmatization would occur; while the actual, demonstrable instances of discrimination and rejection are a third aspect of the situation. Some researchers argue that it is essential for understanding to make distinctions between perceived or 'felt' stigma and experienced or ('actual' or 'enacted') stigma (Scambler and Hopkins, 1988). However, it is not always possible to disentangle the anticipated, perceived, and factual, experiences of people in a stigmatized position, which, in any case, are likely to vary according to gender. As was argued in Chapter 3, socialization for masculine and feminine gender roles influences the actions and situations of adults, while people of different positions in the social structure have different experiences. Analysis of gender differences presents a complex picture and the available research evidence is fragmented.

In certain respects, chronic sick and disabled men are more prone to stigmatization than are women in a like situation. Thus, women are less stigmatized for dependency than are men, because dependency is more compatible with the feminine gender role. Financial dependency on the spouse, a usual consequence of disability, is more stigmatizing for men that for women, because it is unusual or 'different', more of a departure from the accepted husband and wife relationship. Being dependent on others for personal care is distressing for anyone, but for men the more so because dependency is incompatible with the male gender role of being in control.

Men may also suffer more from stigma in particular situations. For example, it was noted in a study of patients treated for long-term 'neurotic' disorders that feelings of stigmatization were expressed by men even more than by women. Neurosis is widely seen as a women's problem, indeed the neurotic woman is a social stereotype. Men found to be neurotic feel themselves ridiculed, as they may well be, for developing a 'woman's' complaint. A works foreman was reported as finding it a huge joke, to be repeated in pubs, that an adult, burly, male job-applicant, suffered from anxiety neurosis (Miles, 1988).

However, there are aspects of stigma and rejection that bear more heavily on women than they do on men. Patterns of social support make the experience of rejection by the social network a more serious problem for women than for men. Women rely a great deal on their friends and wider kin group for support and less so on their husbands. If rejection by network members is experienced, there is nowhere to turn. Men, relying mostly on their wives for support, are less hard hit when friends, relatives and colleagues turn aside.

Rejection by the kin group, then, is especially painful for women. Studies of stigma associated with chronic illness (for example, Hopper, 1981, on diabetes) have found that strong stigmatization can occur in familial relationships, because it is here that problems connected with the illness become most apparent. However, the cultural expectation that families will stand by each other is strong and women are the more hurt when encountering rejection from their mothers, and from female relations who had appeared close to them:

> My Mum has changed, she cannot accept that I am mental, she doesn't want to know.

> My sister-in-law doesn't want me near her children in case I hurt them or go funny, so I don't go there any more.

Women relate such experiences with much pain and hurt (Miles, 1988, p. 73). An attractive-looking undergraduate student, who moved about the campus very competently in a wheelchair, once told the story that she had visited her mother on an occasion when her sister's two young children were staying in the house. When her sister learnt that the children played with her she was horrified: she wanted to spare her children from the sight and knowledge of disability, and accused the mother of negligence. The student explained that she came across stigmatization often, but not until then did she think it possible that it could occur within the family. Thus, in cases where it is not antici- pated, the actual experience of stigmatization is a severe blow.

Those who acquire a stigmatizing attribute as adults (unlike those who were born with one) have to adjust or change entirely their habits when interacting with previous and new social contacts. Women, who prior to their misfortune had a seemingly built-in awareness of how to initiate and pursue acquaintanceships have to reconsider, and almost certainly change, their established modes of interaction. Typical is the feeling of inferiority and fear of stigma: it is better to wait for others to initiate social relations, to wait until old friends choose to come and to withdraw from intercourse with those who appear hesitant and uncer- tain. Diseases which are unpredictable, which may suddenly manifest themselves, are especially handicapping for social relations. In such cases social interaction cannot be pursued with any confidence, as studies of people with epilepsy and Parkinson's disease testify (Pinder, 1988; Scambler and Hopkins, 1988). Women are usually responsible for the social lives of families: it is frequently the wives who initiate and pursue friendships and contacts. Disabled women put much thought and effort into planning and pursuing social intercourse and are more dependent on their success than are disabled men, who can rely on their wives in this respect.

There are other ways, too, in which women suffer more from stigma. Younger women, suffering from chronic sickness, disability or deform- ity, have to face the additional social disadvantage of being regarded as less valuable and desirable on the 'marriage market'. Many personal accounts by young disabled girls include the cry: 'Who will want to marry me?' The letter written by a 16-year-old girl to 'Miss Lonely Hearts', which is reprinted as a preface to Goffman's book on stigma, well expresses this fear (Goffman, 1963):

> I would like to have boy friends like the other girls...but no boy will take me because I was born without a nose.

Women have felt the need to be considered marriageable throughout history: in the aristocratic marriage market women had to show purity, fertility and 'moral correctness' to be marketable, as the inheritance of putative heirs depended thereon (Turner, 1987). In late twentieth cen- tury society, professional men, and managers and executives in the business world, look for handsome and healthy wives who will help their careers; indeed, wives may also be interviewed when husbands look for high-powered employment. Disabled or chronically sick girls are not contemplated as future wives by men in these situations any more than by working-class men whose need is for hard-working, strong and sturdy wives.

One kind of stigma pursues women through much of their lives and bears resemblance to the stigma of long-term illness and permanent disability. If 'differentness' is a basis of stigma it might seem strange that a condition which affects half of the human race could be held to be stigmatizing: such, however, is the case with menstruation, an off-limits subject even today and regarded as polluting and unclean in various societies at various times. It, and the menopause, are discussed later in this chapter. Another, largely feminine, stigma is that accorded to those whose body shape fails to come up to what might be called the 'Hollywood' standard. The greater the emphasis placed on a lissom figure the more disadvantaged are the flat-chested and the heavy-hipped. Obesity and anorexia are discussed next.

Obesity and anorexia

It has been shown that physical blemishes, disfigurements, and disabilities, are stigmatized in contemporary Western societies, where the 'body beautiful' and personal attractiveness are highly valued. There is nothing new in this idealization of the human form – witness the sculpture of Ancient Greece and Rome, echoed, perhaps, in the screen goddesses of our era. If the ideal is not always attainable, those who are regarded as 'too fat' (increasingly the medical term 'obese' is used) or excessively thin (medically, anorexic) are culturally defined as being outside the accepted size range. This is especially so with women.

Obesity is overwhelmingly a women's problem, bringing with it shame, ridicule and discrimination: the 'fat woman' is a figure of fun. To a certain extent, this applies to fat men as well, but the stigma is considerably greater for women, to whom, in any case, it matters more (Wooley and Wooley, 1979; Wooley et al., 1979; Harris et al., 1982).

What is considered attractive is culturally specific: in different societies, at different times, the culturally desirable body size varies. Being large can be regarded a good thing. U.S. sociologist Emily Mumford writes (Mumford, 1983, p. 148):

> Obesity is and has been valued in some societies. In India, a rajah once received gold, jewels, and precious stones equal to his weight each year. On the ceremonial day, the rajah sat on one side of the scale and gold and 'gifts' were heaped on the other until the scale balanced. Doubtless there were some very fat rajahs at that time. In the south of this country [United States], 'She is fat and sassy' was intended as a compliment.

Being large may suggest that one can afford to live well and not have to work too hard, being thin might suggest the opposite. In early societies fatness in women was taken as an indication of fertility and fat ladies carved out of stone are among the fertility symbols found on prehistoric sites. The idea that plump women are best for breeding is not unknown, even today.

In Western Europe and in the United States, the feminine ideal changed frequently during the eighteenth and nineteenth centuries from a renaissance 'buxomness' to the Victorian 18 inch waist: indeed, even in the early part of the present century 'voluptuousness' found favour and dominant beauty images varied between slimness and curves. Mrs Wallis Simpson (later Duchess of Windsor) remarked, famously, 'No-one can be too rich or too slim', and these widely quoted words led to the dieting and deprivation of a large number of U.S. women of her time (Mumford, 1983).

In recent times, it has become culturally desirable for women to be slender. Stereotypes of attractiveness, associated with the very slim fashion models of the 1960s (such as Jean Shrimpton and Twiggy) have been constantly reaffirmed by the fashion industry. Formerly, interest in fashion and fashion models was the concern of the well-off but today fashionable clothes are available in department stores and are widely displayed on television and in women's magazines. Participation in mass culture has brought pressures on women to watch and imitate models and media personalities (Chernin, 1983; Orbach, 1986), and be slim. In addition, medical advice, also widely available on television and in magazines, stresses that to be slim is to be fit and 'healthy' while fatness is associated with ill-health. Medical views on what constitutes obesity change over time, and there is no real consensus regarding definitions: nevertheless, doctors' advice for 'fat people' is to lose weight.

Obesity is a long-term problem (Cradock, 1969). Most fat women tend to fatness through most of their adult lives, some resign themselves to it, others battle ceaselessly to lose weight, many oscillate between acceptance and dieting. Why is conformity to an 'ideal' body size so important for women and why is 'obesity' stigmatized?

An integral part of socialisation for the feminine gender role is the lesson that women must please men, and in this, physical appearance is important. As visible disfigurements and blemishes reduce women's chances to attract men, so does cultural obesity. To be pleasing to men and to be 'marriageable' have been, traditionally, vital for women: excluded from participation in production, women's economic security depended on men.

Obesity is seen in society as a differentness from the acceptable size, and is negatively evaluated: it is associated with an absence of health and fitness and with unattractiveness. As with other stigmatized conditions, several negative characteristics are assigned to the obese: amongst them lack of self-discipline and greed. In an imaginative study, photographs of obese and slim girls were shown to adolescent girls, together with statements purportedly made by the person in the photograph. Responses showed that obese girls were rated as less likable than slim girls by the adolescent female respondents, except where the obese girl of the photograph offered an 'excuse' for her fatness (De Jong, 1980). The obese woman is associated with being 'out of control', and the unrestrained, undisciplined body is associated with general lack of control and laxity (Turner, 1987).

Continuing pressure from the fashion industry, the diet industry and the media, reinforce the stigma of obesity. Fat women are not seen in fashion shows and magazine pictures, and fashion shops seldom cater for the larger women who is apt to experience shame and ridicule when searching for clothes which fit. The diet and slimming trade pushes an increasing range of products aimed at weight reduction; health farms flourish. The message is constantly reaffirmed: health = slimness = happiness. Susie Orbach, arguing that 'fat is a feminist issue', says that 'success, beauty, wealth, love, sexuality and happiness are promoted as attached to and depending on slimness' (Orbach, 1978, p. 25). Women's magazines, whether aimed at higher or lower social-class readers, regularly carry features on how to lose weight, how to avoid food temptations, and how to achieve and keep the perfect figure.

The message from television is less clear-cut. Anne Karpf writes that (Karpf, 1988, p. 203)

> while the documentaries were crowded with health educators spurning fat and extolling fibre, American prime-time drama, it seemed, was full of people doing the opposite. Soap characters scoff puddings and sugary food, snack between meals, eat on the go, and to reward or punish themselves. Yet in spite of all this, they rarely get fat.

Thus, the current cult of slimness, constantly promulgated and medically approved, induces in the fat woman a sense of stigma in public situations (Wiles, 1990):

> I take up too much room on the bus, and, in the dress shop, 'I can't bear to stand in front of the mirror.'

Obesity is not distributed evenly across the population, the lower social classes having a disproportionately high number of obese women. Unlike those societies quoted earlier, where wealth and a full figure are equated, in Western countries the better-off have the desirable slim appearance. There may be several reasons for this: 'slimming food' and other products of the 'diet industry' are expensive; cooking slimming-meals takes more time, thought and energy than does the preparation of 'convenience' or 'fast' food. Working-class women may want to slim as much as middle-class women, but are more hard-pressed for time, money and energy. Many of the exercises which aid slimming are organized by sports clubs and health centres which are more popular with middle-class women, who are also likely to have more leisure.

In a society where the emphasis is on slimness and where fat women are stigmatized, why is 'excessive thinness' a problem for women? In fact, dieting and deprivation carried beyond a certain point result in an emaciated body, disturbed menstruation, and consequent stigma. Wallis Simpson was wrong when she said that no-one can be too thin: she spoke in social terms, meaning that very thin women are attractive. But body size can be 'too thin' as well as 'too fat', bringing negative evaluations; the anorexic woman is regarded as unattractive and is disapproved of.

Anorexia, like other conditions categorized by medicine as 'neurotic disorder' (e.g. depression and anxiety), may be long-term with anorexic women finding themselves stigmatized for their unattractive, unfeminine, body size, for years. It is impossible to define the borderline between slimness and emaciation: as the ideal shape becomes thinner, the dividing line shifts. Many of the writers on anorexia define it in terms other than body-weight; for example, Susie Orbach says in the Introduction to her book *Hunger Strike* (Orbach, 1986, p. 13):

I use anorexia in its broadest possible sense to describe those women who are invested in not eating and have become scared of food and what it can do to them.

Women regarded as obese or anorexic are, typically, held responsible for their condition. The view of friends, relatives, and health professionals, is that individuals are able to regulate the volume of food they eat, and that it is reprehensible to eat too much or too little. Seekers of support often find stigma and rejection instead.

The obese and anorexic conditions and the resulting stigma, present a complex picture. Unlike other stigmatized conditions, it is possible that, to some women, obesity or anorexia is viewed as a form of protest against the social situation of women, exactly because these conditions are stigmatized as 'unfeminine'. Feminist writers have argued that obesity and anorexia are consequences of women's position in society; that women are caught in contradictory expectations regarding their beauty and social value, and that confusing social requirements result in women's ambivalent attitudes to food, eating and body size

(Chernin, 1983). Women are expected to prepare food as an act of love and caring, but not to eat it. According to Ann Oakley (Oakley, 1982, p. 84)

> femininity has traditionally meant the denial or suppression of all physical appetite. Neither sexuality nor food must be eagerly desired, or the feminine standard (passive sexuality, physical thinness) will be transgressed.

It is possible that at least part of the reason why obese and anorexic women alike, eat in ways which result in having bodies deemed un-attractive, is that they do not want to conform to prescribed standards of femininity. Such conduct is a method of escape from the difficulties placed on women by a society shaped by gender inequalities. Bryan Turner argues (Turner, 1987, p. 107)

> anorexia in the twentieth century, like hysteria in the nineteenth century, is expressive of the political limitations on women within a society characterized by inequality between the sexes.

Not to wish to appear attractive to men, is the rejection of a social situation in which women are dependent on pleasing men. In this light, the very stigma that obesity and anorexia bring about serves as a protest.

Menstruation and menopause

The vexed question of whether to regard menstruation, and the dis-comforts surrounding it, as health or illness was discussed in Chapter 2. The problems of menstruation may be regarded as short term, on the grounds that they disappear in a few days, or long term, since they recur every month over a period of 40 years.

The stigma of menstruation is a peculiar kind of stigma: instead of some women being singled out for stigmatization, (as in the case of those with obesity, disability or depression), all women are stigmatized for a few days each month, some more, some less, according to situational and cultural factors. As with, for example, obese or disabled women, menstruating women are viewed negatively, ridiculed, shamed, and subjected to discrimination. They are not held respon-sible for their condition but they are held responsible for their be-haviour while it lasts.

Menstruating women are regarded as unclean in many different cultures, and are required to withdraw from public places, or at least to hide signs of their menstruation (Skultans, 1970). Women, talking about their experiences, often refer to being made to feel dirty. For example, U.S. women in Emily Martin's study (Martin, 1989, p. 93) said

... made me feel like 'Oh, my God, I'm dirty or something'; 'people make you feel bad, especially men. They think that you are dirty when you have your period'; 'something I've had to try to deal with, that I'm not dirty, that I don't stink and smell. It can work against you'.

Stigmatizing menstruating women as 'dirty' leads to shame and embarrassment, feelings also induced by male jokes and ribald stories. Like other very stigmatizing conditions (e.g. mental illness) menstruation is often referred to in derogatory and insulting terms; indeed, an exceptionally wide range of stigma terms are used in the English language. Sophie Laws (1985, p. 18), in a study in England, found that

among boys, the most common form of joking is about sanitary towels, calling them 'jam rags', or variants of this – 'jam roll', 'jam sandwich', etc.

Adult men joked more about sexual access, referring to men who 'picked the wrong one' and to girls with 'sunny periods' (Laws, 1985). American men, too, frequently use terms which express disgust ('blood and sand'; 'ketchup'; 'dirty red') or sexual unavailability ('ice-box' and 'manhole covers'). A current Americanism is 'OTR' meaning 'on-the-rag' (Shuttle and Redgrove, 1986). (This variety of jokey/insulting terms bears resemblance to the stigmatizing terms used concerning the mentally ill, e.g. 'fruit-cake', 'nut-case', 'potty' and 'round the bend'). A consequence of stigma is that menstruating women feel ashamed, try hard to conceal any sign of their condition from public view, and in many cases think of themselves as 'dirty' (Scambler and Scambler, 1985). Another consequence is discrimination: menstruating women are regarded as moody, bad tempered, and unreliable, and with this condition recurring for several days in every month, the result is that men regard women as generally unsuitable for positions of power and responsibility. Even the office and the factory floor are more suitable places for men than for women whose functions may occasionally incapacitate them. American writer Emily Martin (Martin, 1989, pp. 99–100) thinks that women should

ask why the outside world does not legitimate the functions of women's bodies ... and why the workplace in this country is so incompatible with women's reproductive roles.

Women during the years of menopause are similarly shamed and devalued; they, too, try to conceal the condition which, although regarded as 'natural', is stigmatized. The visible physical indications of the menopause, mainly the 'hot flushes', are deeply stigmatizing. Women often talk about the 'embarrassment' of having hot flushes in public places. In research interviews, women tend to refer to such embarrassment as if this were a 'natural' response, not needing to be explained; indeed, few women are able to put into words their reasons for feeling embarrassed. Martin (1989, p. 168) reports:

> I can remember being very embarrassed talking with a fellow worker and my face turned very red ... I was sure that it was written all over my face what the cause of that redness was and there was nothing for me to be blushing about, nothing in the conversation that was embarrassing, so I remember those little embarrassing episodes ... just praying that he didn't notice it.

And Phillips and Rakusen, (1978, p. 518):

> I also had hot flushes several times a week for almost six months. I didn't get as embarrassed as some of my friends who also had hot flushes, but I found the heat-wave sensation most uncomfortable.

Martin again (1989, p. 169):

> I am active, I am busy, and thinking. That is when it would happen. But if you are talking to someone eyeball to eyeball and you are trying to convince them and sell them on something and you start sweating, they look at you ... Yes, I was embarrassed.

Women are especially ashamed of hot flushes when these occur in the workplace. According to Emily Martin (Martin, 1989, p. 168), this is partly because hot flushes are outward signs, publicly displayed, of inner bodily processes of the reproductive system which are supposed to be kept private, and partly because

> they reveal indisputably that one is a woman and a woman of a certain age, in situations where one is projecting the aspect of self as colleague, fellow worker, leader, or reliable functionary.

Several negative characteristics are attributed to menopausal women: they are regarded as unreliable, lacking stamina, and as being 'out-of-control', irrational and unbalanced (Oakley, 1982). Such negative images are fostered by health professionals who point out that menopausal 'hormone imbalance' is likely to lead to 'psychological imbalance'. It seems that the cessation of menstruation, like menstruation itself, labels women as unpredictable; indeed, it is part of the feminist writers' argument that women in Western societies are defined in terms of their reproductive system.

The cultural roots of the stigma attached to the menopause are quite deep. The menopause signals the end of a woman's ability to bear children. In cultures where child-bearing and child-rearing are considered to be the main contributions of women to society, menopause implies the end of usefulness (Morsy, 1978; Currer, 1986). ('Barren' women in such cultures are similarly stigmatized.) In late twentieth century Western societies, traditional views of women's usefulness as child-bearers struggle with feminist views of women as main contributors elsewhere than in the sphere of reproduction: consequently there are two clashing views of the menopause: as 'obsolescence' and as 'renewal' (Kaufert, 1982). Medical textbooks describe the menopause in language indicating the former: it is the 'death of the woman in the woman'; the 'breakdown of the system'; 'a state where 'functions fail'; 'ovaries regress', and 'genital organs gradually atrophy' (Ehrenreich and English, 1979, p. 111; Martin, 1989, p. 42). Medical men (the authors of textbooks have been almost all men) are not the only 'experts' using such language. According to Patricia Kaufert (Kaufert, 1982, p. 160)

> The classical Freudians, as represented by Deutsch (1944), defined the menopause as obsolescence; it meant that woman had 'reached her natural end – her partial death – as servant to the species'. From Deutsch's perspective, the menopause can only be seen as loss; loss of fertility, loss of femininity, loss of meaning in a woman's life.

Contemporary physicians and psychiatrists also stress the loss aspect in women's lives; they talk of the 'empty nest' (i.e. when grown-up children have left home) and the loss of the mothering and home-making function of women, their very 'femininity'.

Linked to all this is another kind of loss: physical attractiveness. In Western societies feminine good looks are important values (as discussed previously) and so is youth. Indeed, some would argue that in our 'youth-orientated culture' very negative attitudes to ageing prevail and the abilities of older women are minimized, while 'youthfulness is falsely glorified' (Phillips and Rakusen, 1978).

Older women's groups often unwittingly reinforce the emphasis on youth by advising menopausal women how to 'preserve' their physical attractiveness, conceal their age, and maintain the appearance of youth. Cosmetic and beauty industries relay the same message in advertizing their products: there is no need to show wrinkles or grey hair.

Thus, the stigma of the menopause is rooted in notions of women losing their usefulness, good looks and youth as well as in the notion of the menopause bringing psychological imbalance, i.e. irritability, unreliability and other indicators of a less valuable person.

It is interesting to note that the negative attributes of the menopause are more feared by younger women (anticipated stigma) than the reality, as described by older women, would warrant. Studies of women's attitudes show that young women anticipate this phase of women's lives with apprehension, expecting many problems, while many menopausal women say that they experienced few physical problems and their bad experiences were mainly social (Martin, 1989). The Boston Women's Health Book Collective surveyed nearly 500 women in the United States; they write (Phillips and Rakusen, 1978, p. 530).

> In general, younger women were more fearful and felt more negative about menopause. Older women, especially post-menopausal women, were more matter of fact. This suggests that younger women tend to have a distorted view of the menopausal experience, anticipating it as much worse than it usually turns out to be. Is this because of all the myths about menopause that surrounds it? Is it because younger women especially fear our society's attitude towards ageing women?

Strategems of coping with relationships

People who have to live with long-term stigmatizing health problems develop their own ways, or 'stratagems' of coping with social interaction. There are a number of possibilities depending on the nature of the problem and on the immediate social situation.

One stratagem is concealment: the stigmatizing condition is hidden away from as many relatives, friends and colleagues as possible and interaction is conducted as though the condition was not present. This stratagem is available only to those whose condition is not readily apparent, e.g. carriers of the AIDs virus HIV bear no distinguishing signs. As previously discussed, social etiquette requires women to conceal evidence of menstruation while the menopause can be denied even in response to questioning (Laws, 1985; Kaufert and Gilbert, 1986a). Many women will choose to conceal a psychiatric diagnosis and the subsequent treatment. Such decisions are made in concrete situations; for example, the general consensus among women being treated for depression, agoraphobia and other 'neurotic' problems is that the condition should be concealed from prospective employers wherever possible; that a history of psychiatric treatment should not be volunteered ('that would be stupid' and 'I would never risk it') although may be admitted in the face of a direct question ('I wouldn't say unless there was a question on the form. I would say it then'; 'Not on the application form, wouldn't stand a chance, I might tell at the interview') (Miles, 1988, p. 82).

Other situations are less clear-cut, and whether to conceal or not has to be decided again and again with each relationship. A sympathetic attitude from a friend can lead to confidences, a hostile reception from another can bring about further concealment. The main problem with this stratagem is that what is concealed may come to light; anxiety over possible discovery may be as bad as the reality of negative responses from colleagues or friends. A woman in the early stages of multiple sclerosis, with no visible signs, said in a research interview that she did not intend to 'admit' the diagnosis to anyone unless she found that she could not 'stand the strain' of maintaining relationships with colleagues and neighbours 'based on a lie' (Miles, 1984). Concealment is a specially precarious stratagem for those whose disease is inherently unpredictable, with symptoms which may appear suddenly. Thus, in Ruth Pinder's study (Pinder, 1988, pp. 76–77), a woman with Parkinson's disease explained that she organized her working life around the management and "covering" of symptoms, although foot spasms occurred periodically, and stretched her ability to conceal them to the limit:

> I arrange things at the office, appointments, when I know I'm going to be in an 'on' situation, which is why I put Thursday night for the interview because I don't work Friday mornings...It happened once [foot spasms] when I was taking a property on and I didn't know what to do, because he didn't know and I was trying to carry on a conversation and trying to control it from the inside. I can't talk and control it at the same time. You need to be very careful not to have too long a day and take an outside appointment at the end of the day. It's at the end of the day when it happens.

In spite of the problems of management, and worries over disclosure, concealment is to many women a viable stratagem, enabling them to lead a near-normal life and keep their jobs. In fact, this appears to be a favoured situation for both male and female sufferers from a variety of conditions, such as the mentally ill (Brockman *et al.*, 1979), the epileptic (Scambler and Hopkins, 1988), patients with skin diseases (Jobling, 1988) and the deaf (Becker, 1981).

Another stratagem is 'normalization'. Without trying to hide the condition, the individual may attempt to minimize its impact on social relations, to make light of its importance, and to deny that the disease or disability is a potential barrier to ordinary social interaction. Fred Davis describes normalization, in his study of children disabled by polio, as a stratagem by which polio patients are trying to say, 'Though

I may appear different, I really am not. Not only do I think of myself as normal, but others think of me as normal too.' (Davis, 1963, p. 140).

The stratagem of normalization is more likely to be successful in cases of moderately incapacitating conditions than in very severe ones; indeed, for those needing constant help with personal daily care, this stratagem is not available.

When the condition is such as to necessitate the giving up of employment, women have a better chance than men of successfully normalizing other social relationships. A study of multiple sclerosis patients revealed that unemployed female patients found it easier to achieve normal or near-normal relationships than did their male counterparts. Of course, the constant presence of a wife in the home accords more easily with normal expectations than does the constant presence of a husband, sick or not (Miles, 1979, p. 323):

> Mrs Murray had multiple sclerosis quite severely, but she had, against advice, resisted the wheelchair solution as she was able to walk a few steps in the house by holding on to the furniture. Details of daily routine showed the constant presence of helpers and visitors. Relatives visited them, a sister and sister-in-law lived nearby and came in to give a hand and to gossip; neighbours called in frequently and their son brought his friends home...The house was cheerfully crowded, very untidy and lively. Both husband and wife asserted that the illness made no difference to their social life.

Blaxter (1976), studying patients with different disabling conditions, recorded a similar pattern of women adapting more readily than men in a like situation. An unemployed disabled man is unlikely to pursue normalization successfully: work, the centre pin of his life, is knocked away, relationships with workmates are discontinued, and the setting of socialization, pub or club, no longer welcoming.

The stratagem of normalization depends on the willingness of the healthy members of the social network to go along with it. The disabled housewife is more likely to be able to pursue previous social relations in and around the domestic sphere than is the disabled man to do likewise in the arenas of work and sport.

'Disassociation' is another stratagem of coping with relationships. Some disabled, sick or deformed people feel that their condition acts as a barrier to ordinary social interaction and so they withdraw from involvement with the social group around them. Typically, individuals who feel that their condition is much stigmatized opt for this course, not wanting to expose themselves to snubs, rejections, or ridicule. Women with visible disfigurements, even the 'grossly obese', may withdraw from social activity, feeling that their appearance is off-putting if not repulsive; those with visible scars, burn-marks and skin diseases often seek to hide themselves from the public gaze (Orbach, 1978). It will be apparent that disassociation is not so much a way of coping with relationships but their abandonment, less of a stratagem than a surrender.

Finally, there is the stratagem, advocated by political activists, of fighting the healthy, non-stigmatized social group for the rights of the stigmatized to equal treatment. At the level of personal relationships, this stratagem means refusal to accept a definition of oneself as 'deformed' or 'generally disabled' or otherwise stigmatized; refusal to retreat, withdraw, or to conceal the disability or sickness, but on the contrary to demand acceptance on equal terms, to persuade or force other people to change the ways in which they talk or act concerning the disabled or otherwise stigmatized. In other words, the strategy is to 'tough it out'.

Women who are feminists and involved in the Women's Health Movement are specially likely to opt for this stratagem, but it is by no means limited to them. Thus, a woman talking about her way of dealing with hot flushes at her workplace (Martin, 1989, p. 169):

> I think that in the beginning I used to say that I was hot and I can't take the heat, or I just had a cold. And after a while I would say that I was going through my menopause, damn it. That is what you should say. That shuts them up fast. Especially a man...Yes, well, let them be embarrassed. I was tired of being embarrassed.

It is difficult to pursue this stratagem alone, without support; women, by organizing themselves into groups, find it easier to face the stigmatizers: thus, fat women who form groups to resist ridicule, shame and discrimination, find confidence to say, 'I am fat, happy, and not ashamed'.

Stratagems devised for conducting relationships are seldom sustainable; rather do they need constantly to be modified in the face of new acquaintances and new situations. Studies of the disabled, the long-term sick, and the disfigured, report an oscillating pattern of disclosure and concealment, of demanding rights and of retreating rebuffed. The responses of healthy, able-bodied groups, potential helpers and potential stigmatizers, have constantly to be evaluated and stratagems reconsidered (Doll *et al.*, 1976; Ablon, 1981; Harris and Smith, 1983). Indeed, it can be stated positively that ambiguity and uncertainty lie at the core of the social situation of the long-term sick and the disabled.

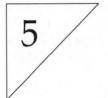

Women in medicine

Division of labour in health work

The second half of the twentieth century has seen a large increase in the numbers of people engaged in health occupations in Western industrial societies. There is constant pressure for further expansion of these occupations as greater affluence makes possible increased investment in better health. The conquest of 'old' diseases such as smallpox and tuberculosis encourages the belief that all disease is conquerable, given enough resources, while new problems, AIDS, drug abuse, etc., along with new scientific discoveries, bring with them a demand for new and expanded services.

Throughout history there have been people involved in healing and caring for the sick. Now, rapid advances in medicine and the ever-increasing expectation of good health have brought into existence a growing number of specialists offering a wide range of health care services. Healing occupations of long tradition, such as doctors and nurses, have been joined by many new ones, indeed, on-going medical advances coupled with the large-scale organization of health care has led to a proliferation of specialist occupational groups, all seeking recognition; all demanding new training programmes. To these must be added the large labour force necessary for the running and maintenances of modern hospitals.

Thus, the practice of healing operates within the framework of a complex division of labour, a term which, in the context of health care, refers to the ways in which the tasks surrounding the care and treatment of the sick, the prevention of illness and the furtherance of knowledge to these ends, are shared out among many occupational groups.

Despite differences of approach, the various sociologists who have applied themselves to this division of labour, agree that it is hierarchical in character, some occupations and groups of workers being accorded higher prestige and financial rewards, and wielding more power, than others. An influential sociological analysis was that of Eliot Freidson in the early 1970s for whom the crucial feature of the division of labour in health care was that control over it was exercised by the medical profession, i.e. the doctors. From an historical perspective Freidson traced the emergence of the profession of doctor, describing it as an occupation 'which has gained the exclusive right to practise medicine by virtue of the support of the state and its own occupational organisation' (Freidson, 1975a p. 47). He repeatedly stressed that the doctors, as the dominant profession, were able to control not only their own work, but the work of other occupations allied to the task of healing (p. 48):

What the physician does is a part of a larger technical division of labour and sometimes not a very distinct or generic part. It is the physician's *control* of the division of labour that is distinct. Those occupations falling under his control are called 'paramedical' [original emphasis].

The paramedical occupations referred to includes the qualified nurses, who, at the time of Florence Nightingale and at her insistence, became defined as subordinate to doctors. According to Freidson's account (Freidson, 1975a, p. 61):

Nightingale required that what the nurse did for the patient was a function of what the doctor felt was required for the care of the patient . . . All nursing work flowed from the doctor's orders.

Newer occupations – physiotherapists, medical laboratory technicians, occupational therapists and many others – developed during the twentieth century, at a time when the control of doctors was well established and thus these occupations became 'subordinate' from their beginnings. Freidson allowed that some specialties, e.g. dentistry and optometry, had survived independently, but in the main all of the 'paramedical' qualified skilled occupations were subordinate to doctors. Consequentially, Freidson argued, these occupations were accorded inferior prestige and economic standing and were recruited from lower social classes than were the doctors. Worse, they enjoyed only limited occupational autonomy; they could not independently attract their clientele, but had to rely on referral by doctors. Much of their education and training was spent learning 'medical knowledge' i.e. knowledge of anatomy, physiology, pathology, etc., which the

medical profession had earlier successfully established as being within
its own province; doctors frequently acted not only as teachers but
decision-makers as to the content and volume of 'suitable' knowledge
for students in the paramedical occupations. In this, the purpose of
doctors was to help to train groups of skilled workers who could
eventually take certain tasks, not requiring the full weight of medical
knowledge, off the doctors themselves, thereby lightening their own
load in areas of work they found unattractive. From the doctors' perspective, this seemed a legitimate aim: like captains of ships and of
industry, they needed skilled groups of helpers. From the perspective
of the paramedical occupations, however, the situation was otherwise:
they, to varying extent, wanted to become independent of doctors in
order to be able to develop their own special contributions to health
care in their own ways and in the process to enhance both their
prestige and their economic standing.

Writing about inter-occupational relations in the health services,
Freidson (1975a) argued that functional autonomy, defined as the degree to which work can be carried on independently of organizational
or medical supervision, is a crucial factor in the hierarchy of occupational relationships (pp. 53–54):

> On the whole, the more autonomous the occupation and the
> greater the overlap of its work with that of physicians, the greater
> is the potential for conflict, legal or otherwise ... conflict is
> common, focusing around the question of whether or not non-
> physicians are to be allowed to offer health services independent-
> ly of medical supervision.

In their struggle for autonomy the health occupations can aim to
implement measures which at the same time will improve their standing in society, and in this connection Freidson stressed the importance
of recruitment and training: 'the longer, the more formal and the closer
training is to the university, the higher the position in the division of
labour' (Freidson, 1975a, p. 55). Another important issue in occupational struggles is the 'area of competence'. If the doctors achieved
their dominant position through successfully claiming monopoly over
the core tasks of diagnosis and prescription of treatment, the way
forward for other health occupations might well be to establish
monopoly of practice over their own spheres of health care. As Freidson (p. 66) points out, however, the dilemma facing each of these
occupations is that

> to escape subordination to medical authority, it must find some
> area of work over which it can claim and maintain a monopoly,
> but it must do so in a setting in which the central task *is* healing
> and controlled by medicine. [original emphasis]

During the years which followed Freidson's analysis, the struggle for autonomy and higher economic rewards and prestige continued. 'Paramedical', the term used freely by Freidson to describe the non-medical health occupations became contentious, as seeming to denote their subordinate status, while the alternative 'ancillary to medicine' appeared no better. 'Allied to medicine' and 'supplementary to medicine' are synonyms favoured by some but perhaps the simplest solution is for all these groups to be known as 'health occupations'.

Freidson's analysis of the 1970s has been expanded upon and criticized by more recent writers. Some see the doctors' power as stemming not so much from their control of the health occupations (which is weakening) but from their continued right of access to patients. It is still the case that other health professionals rely overwhelmingly on the doctors for their clientele. Doctors have enhanced their prestige by strengthening their relationship with biochemistry, pharmacology, physics and other sciences, and have maintained their grip on the knowledge base: nursing schools are located in hospitals and the curriculum committees are dominated by doctors. However, the new skilled health occupations are asserting themselves and, with the new-style managers of the health industry, are posing a major challenge to medical dominance (Larkin, 1981; Ovretveit, 1985).

Another criticism of Freidson's analysis of the health labour force is that he paid little attention to issues of class, gender and ethnic origin. Indeed, it is characteristic of the writings of many medical sociologists of the 1960s and 1970s (somewhat less so in the 1980s) that their use of such generic categories as 'doctors', 'patients', and 'nurses', paid scant regard to these and similar issues. Analysis of relationships, personal or occupational, frequently suffered the same failing. It can certainly be argued that any discussion of the division of labour in the health 'industry' lacks sufficiency if class, gender, age and ethnic origin are not taken into account.

An analysis of the health division of labour as part of the structure of the general labour force of modern Western societies, was given by Vincente Navarro, a U.S. Marxist sociologist who argued that the health labour force should be viewed as an integral part of the class structure of capitalist societies (Navarro, 1976).

It is part of Navarro's general critical stance that Freidson neglected to consider, as an integral part of the division of labour in health, the position of the large numbers of unskilled and semi-skilled manual workers involved with the running of large organizations, especially hospitals. According to Navarro's scheme, the important characteristic of this division of labour is that the dominant profession of doctors, together with the top managers and administrators, constitute the upper class of the hierarchy; the qualified, skilled groups of workers, such as the nurses, the various therapists, the radiographers and many of the administrative and technical staff, constitute the middle class and below them are the working class of the health-care industry, namely hospital domestic staff, laundry and catering staff, porters and maintenance workers and many others. As in other areas of the division of labour in developed societies, the hierarchy in health-care is complex and undergoing constant change. The standing and relationship of the various occupations shifts, not merely *vis-à-vis* the dominant doctors, but relative to each other and any analysis of the situation, such as those offered by Freidson and Navarro, risks implying a more static situation than is really the case.

When analysing the position of the health occupations and the relationships between them, attention should be given not only to the nature of the work and the economic and power position of these groups, but also to the class origin of the members of the occupations. There is much evidence of selective recruiting. In the UK, the Todd Report on medical education showed that about 40 per cent of medical students came from families of the professional and executive classes and only 3 per cent from families of semi-skilled and unskilled workers (Royal Commission, 1968). Subsequent, smaller, studies of medical undergraduates reveal little or no change in this pattern. Other studies of the social origins of university students generally confirm that change is slower and on a smaller scale than, perhaps, is generally believed. Medical students, requiring the longest training, put more demands on parental resources than do others; encouragement and financial support come most easily from upper middle-class homes.

Patterns of recruiting into the occupations of nursing, physiotherapy and other skilled health occupations are less well documented. Students in these groups, with some exceptions, receive non-university level education on qualifying courses; colleges of higher education, with less rigorous entrance requirements, frequently draw their students from the lower middle and skilled working classes. The largest group of health workers, the unskilled and semi-skilled labour force engaged in laundries, or catering, or maintenance work, or as porters, drivers, gardeners, etc., are most likely to come from working-class families, but there is very little direct evidence (Doyal, 1983). It is rather the studies of social stratification in the UK that provide the information on which such assumptions can be made.

The class structure of the UK health labour force, then, has an upper, middle and working class, a pattern which has also been demonstrated by writers working in the United States, Australia, Canada and elsewhere.

The gender division of labour in health work

Most writers, in discussing the division of labour in health work, make reference to the unequal distribution of women in the hierarchy. Often such references are scanty, even dismissive, implying that gender divisions are of little consequence. However, in recent years thorough analyses of the role of gender in health work have been carried out by a number of feminist writers who offer fresh information on the history of healing and healers (Davies, 1980; Mitchell and Oakley, 1986; Stacey, 1988) and on the role of gender relations in health work (Game and Pringle, 1984). Sociological analyses of work settings in hospitals, general practice and community care have also shed new light on gender relations in the field of health (Cartwright and Anderson, 1981; Jefferys and Sachs, 1983). In addition, attention has been focused on the role of gender in health work carried out in the home (Graham, 1983; Finch and Groves, 1983).

In many Western countries, during most of the twentieth century, the majority of doctors have been men, and the majority of both skilled and unskilled health workers have been women. The task of current sociological studies of sex distribution in the health labour force is to explain the affect of this situation on the work and on the relations of workers, and to explain why and how and with what consequences changes may occur.

In the British National Health Service, 75 per cent of the workers are women but their distribution in the hierarchy is very unequal. Only about 20 per cent of doctors in Britain are women as against more than 90 per cent of the nurses; other non-medical occupations, such as physiotherapy and occupational therapy are similarly constituted. Three-quarters of the semi-skilled and unskilled manual workers in the health labour force are women, most of them employed part-time.

In England, the total number of hospital doctors, in 1986, was 36305 of whom 8868 were female. At the same time women comprised some 18 per cent of general practitioners. These figures reveal that a major change has taken place since the early part of the century, when women formed only 3–5 per cent of all doctors.

Of the various occupational relationships in the area of health, that of male doctor–female nurse has received most attention possibly because it has longer roots than relationships between more recently emerged occupations. Many writers have pointed out the 'family symbolism' in the relationship: doctor as father, nurse as mother and the patient as child, relations between them reflecting relationships in the domestic sphere (Game and Pringle, 1984). The Nightingale tradition in nursing emphasized obedience to doctors, and the valued qualities of patience, unselfishness, devotion and quietness in nurses. Certainly, nurses in that tradition were not encouraged to consider themselves as 'colleagues' of doctors – they were there to help and assist. The parallel between the Nightingale tradition and the Victorian family tradition seems strong: the father-doctor was responsible for the well-being of the family; he made the decisions and expected, and received, help, support and acquiescence from the mother-nurse. Of course, both doctors and nurses worked within their own hierarchical systems: the nurses had their own strictly-defined hierarchy with the matron wielding authority over 'her' staff; among doctors, junior and senior, each had an understood place in the pecking order. However, on the hospital ward, where the 'doctor–nurse game' is most frequently played out, the power relationship throughout the century, and, with modifications, even today, can be seen as a reflection of family relations. In Leeson and Gray's (1978) description (pp. 62–63):

> the doctor–nurse–patient relationship in and out of hospital is largely based on that which usually obtains at ward level. That relationship mirrors the stereotype of the bourgeois family where father dominates and performs the role of decision-taker and protector whilst mother's role is passive, consisting of servicing activities and carrying out the wishes of father. The child's role is subordinate, her rights are limited, she is serviced by mother, her needs are interpreted by mother to father and her daily performance related to father by mother.

On the ward, the consultant is accompanied by the nurse who tells him what she has been doing while he has been away; the doctor, having examined the patient, leaves instructions with the nurse as to what she must do. The family analogy has also the implication that doctor and nurse, like father and mother, should stick together for the sake of their dependants and the good reputation of the organization (Leeson and Gray, 1978).

The sex stereotyping of doctors and nurses in Britain and North America is very strong and is acquired in childhood. Studies of pre-school and early school-age children show the extent to which sex stereotyping is learnt from adults through toys, games, reading material and the mass media. For example, Goodman (1974) conducted a pre-Christmas participant observation study in a large U.S. store's toy department and found adult buyers had quite rigid gender-related preconceptions about the appropriate toys for children over two years of age. When buying costumes for children, boys received highway patrol, astronauts and Indian chief outfits, but nurse costumes were always for girls, together with those simulating brides and ballerinas. Girls received nursing kit, but never doctoring kit (Goodman, 1974). Several other studies have demonstrated that books, comics and magazines for boys and girls are gender-differentiated, that segregated gender-specific adult roles are learned in early reading schemes, that gender stereotyping in television children's programmes is marked, and that parental encouragement and approval of games and plays are sex-orientated (Lobban, 1978; Walkerdine, 1984). The role of nurse in childhood games is for girls, and the role of doctor is for boys; that is the clear message.

In addition to toys and games and the mass media all relaying the same message, real-life experiences of children also confirm the image of the nurse as female. The child's first nurse is usually its mother who nurses it through all the ailments of childhood. Fathers take little or no part in the bedside care of sick children (albeit for reasons which may seem adequate) and this experience confirms the notion that nurse equals mother or, at least, a female adult (Maclean, 1974).

The sex stereotyping of the more recent and largely female health occupations is not as strong as that of nurse and doctor. There is no study to show whether, for example, physiotherapists, occupational therapists and speech therapists are represented in children's toys, games or comics, but the likelihood is that they are not. Even adults hardly know what to expect when first encountering these newer health workers; indeed they are often uncertain as to who they are and what they do (Miles, 1988; Martin, 1989). However, in hospitals, the doctor–nurse game is often replicated by doctor–therapist: the message conveyed to patients is that the doctor (usually male) is in charge, gives instructions and expects compliance.

Why is it that in the United States, UK, Australia and other Western countries, the sex stereotyping of doctors and nurses is so resistant to change? Cultural preconceptions of the essential qualities of male and female have often been cited in attempts to explain the reasons for these occupations being dominated by men and by women, respectively. The woman 'cares' for her unborn child, suckles and comforts the baby and so is seen as possessing innate attributes which enable her to nurture and be kind to the weak and dependent, making her the obvious candidate for nursing the sick and other forms of care. Men are believed to have a natural aptitude for things scientific and technological, characteristics which fit very well the popular image of medicine which, accordingly, is seen as man's work. Cultural assumptions are made not just about the difference between male and female qualities but also about the respective nature of medical and nursing work. Such assumptions may be fallacious, and it is important to bear in mind that cultural preconceptions may well differ as between different societies and at different times. What is seen today as established practice according to which doctors are male and nurses are female, is actually of quite recent origin.

From ancient times women have been involved in the tasks of di-
agnosing and treating illness and caring for the sick. Women elders of
primitive groups (as, indeed, of some societies today) advised younger
members on the avoidance of illness and its treatments. Women who
had themselves borne children assisted others in parturition (Mead,
1935; Ehrenreich and English, 1979; Marieskind, 1980). According to
Versluysen, (1980), drawing on the studies of historians,

> women's past medical work had been varied and extensive in
> scope and had involved women of all social classes, from the
> wise women skilled in the use of herbs and ointments, to the
> chatelaine in her castle, and the woman selling her skills as
> physician and surgeon in the open market.

And he goes on further that

> before the late seventeenth century, the male impact on the
> everyday healing experience of most people was minimal.

In many societies, past and present, 'wise women' have possessed
specialized knowledge of herbal and other remedies for preventing and
treating sickness. This kind of knowledge, based on observations,
experimentations, and handed down from one generation to another,
often now called 'old-wives' tales', frequently had a sound empirical
basis (Graham and Oakley, 1986).

Many historians have documented the rise of scientific Western
medicine, and with it the separation of the healing from the caring of
the sick (Versluysen, 1980). In the course of this separation the new
and increasingly powerful scientific medicine became a male preserve.
During the nineteenth and early twentieth centuries in Britain and the
United States the exclusion of women from the medical profession
became all but total, while the occupation of nursing became almost
entirely a female preserve. As Leeson and Gray (1978) observed, 'his-
torically, the notion that only men can make suitable doctors is a
relatively new idea and in very few places has general medical care
ever been provided by men'. They say also (p. 20) that the 'currently
accepted wisdom of Western Europe and North America that a doctor's
duties are more suitably performed by men than by women is so
patent an aberration, local in time and place'.

In Eastern Europe the situation has developed quite differently and
today the medical profession in the Soviet Union, Hungary and
Czechoslovakia is largely a female one. In these countries between 70
and 85 per cent of the doctors are women.

Descriptions of the sex stereotyping of occupations and of expectations as to how doctors, nurses and other therapists relate to each
other, can be over-simplified. The reality is more complex, and certain-

ly not static. Complexities arise from the improvement in the standing and independence of the various health occupations, the possibility that medical dominance is declining, the boundary disputes which constantly arise between occupational groups, from variations in the doctor–nurse relationships and, not the least from the recruitment of more women to the medical profession and more men to nursing.

The subordination of female nurses to the authority and control of male physicians is neither so complete nor so unproblematic as the early work of writers such as Freidson implied. Indeed, Freidson himself, in a later work, painted a more complex picture (Freidson, 1986). For example, in situations where the nurse has more experience than the doctor with whom she works, or where the nurse's status in her own hierarchy is considerably higher than that of the doctor in his, or when the indigenous nurse works with a relatively new-come foreign doctor, their relationships may stray from the stereotype. A study by David Hughes, undertaken in the casualty department of a British hospital, showed that experienced nurses volunteered, or were asked to give, advice to junior doctors and locums (Hughes, 1988). Doctors there were either recently qualified with short-term appointments, or older male general practitioners with little recent casualty experience. Some doctors were recent immigrants, not yet at home with the English language and culture. The nurses on the other hand were established, experienced staff. According to Hughes, his study showed *not* that 'medical dominance breaks down completely, but that various work exigencies mean that its impact is considerably weakened in many informal interactions' (p. 16). Other recent writers have found similar complexities in nurse–doctor relationships (Dingwall *et al.*, 1983). Thus, even the most stereotypical relationship, that between doctor and nurse, may empirically differ from the cultural expectation of their respective dominance and submissiveness. Disputes between the medical profession and developing health occupations, struggling for autonomy and independence, have been well documented by recent studies (Larkin, 1981; Ovretveit, 1985). These and other writers differ as to the extent by which medical dominance is accordingly reduced; but the perceived picture of doctors as occupying the highest position in a hierarchical division of labour remains largely intact.

Preparing for medical work

'One of the problems of medical education today is to contain the ever-swelling tide of new knowledge within the confines of the curriculum' (*Everyman's Encyclopaedia*, 1967 edition). If that was the situation at the time when this sentence was written, then it is very much more so today and medical students face stiff and prolonged educational programmes embracing other disciplines besides that of medicine.

Constant broadening of the knowledge base of virtually every subject bearing on healing and health care has meant that the education of students for membership of the health-related occupations is likewise increasingly prolonged and demanding. Students in schools of physiotherapy, occupational therapy, nursing and elsewhere are expected to undergo stiff educational programmes, drawing on various disciplines to attain increasingly higher levels, as these occupations strive to reach parity of esteem with doctors and scientists. How relevant are gender issues in the education of students? How do women fare in the various educational establishments?

During most of the twentieth century women constituted a small percentage of medical students in Western countries where, as we have seen, the profession was overwhelmingly a male preserve. In the United States, the number of women in medical schools remained at around 6–8 per cent between 1914 and the 1960s, except that during World War II numbers rose to more than 10 per cent before slipping back to 5.5 per cent by 1960 (Mumford, 1983, p. 270). From the end of the 1960s the situation started to change until, by 1979, 23 per cent of graduating medical students were women. The position in Britain mirrored the U.S. experience in that from small beginnings in the early part of the century, no significant increase in the number of women entering medical schools was recorded until well into the 1960s. Then, in both countries, sex discrimination legislation began to make an impact so that today the numbers of male and female students in medical schools are broadly in balance.

That women in medical schools are no longer in a minority makes it the more interesting to observe that they often behave as though they were. Like female students in engineering and other numerically male-dominated university courses, they feel a greater sense of insecurity than do the men students; they feel that they must try harder to show that they are equal to the demands made upon students, demonstrate a greater commitment to the cultural norms of the institution and, above all, obtain higher results in order to gain status similar to the men (Rosenblatt and Kirk, 1982; Lorber, 1984; Grossman *et al.*, 1987). The writer's own conversations with female medical students indicate that for them this situation is part and parcel of medical-school life.

The reasons for the somewhat diffident attitudes adopted by female medical students can be located in the sex stereotyping of doctors and nurses earlier discussed. This stereotyping, absorbed in childhood, is likely to be reinforced in adolescence and adulthood. TV soap operas, set in hospitals, all too often lend substance to the theme of dominant doctor/subservient nurse. Parents and teachers, themselves influenced by prevailing prejudice, are likely to discourage the aspirant female doctor. Once in medical school, the female student will observe that among the academic and clinical teaching staff her sex is grossly unrepresented especially in the higher echelons of power. Notwithstanding the new-found emancipation of women, their minority status in terms of authority, position and power in medical schools remains a fact of life.

Any expectation that increasing the numbers of women students would result in their greater acceptance by male colleagues and teachers has yet to be borne out. Indeed, Lorber (1984) found that in U.S. medical schools, the reverse was almost the case, that their increase from a few to a substantial minority not only failed to result in better integration, but that they received even less support and encouragement from male teachers. However, long-held attitudes are slow to change and it must still be the hope that as equal sex distribution of medical students becomes established through generations of graduates, integration will follow and that, as ever more female students become doctors, the lingering resentment of women in the profession of medicine will finally be eradicated. But this ideal state of affairs is still in the future; the present reality is different.

As students enter medical schools they begin a process of education and socialization during which they learn, not only the formal subjects of the curriculum, but also the values and beliefs of the medical profession. Two studies of U.S. medical schools, now regarded as 'classic', were carried out during the 1950s, namely *The Student Physician* (Merton *et al.*, 1957) at Harvard and *Boys in White* (Becker *et al.*, 1961) in Chicago. These studies suggested that besides acquiring medical knowledge and skills, students also learnt from their teachers how to play the 'role of the doctor' by absorbing their beliefs, expectations and norms. The mechanism by which such socialization takes place has engendered much sociological discussion, some emphasizing the importance of the medical curriculum, others the structural factors of work organization and work settings, others again, the influence of role models, interactive processes and personal values (Freidson, 1975a). Less attention has been paid to the possibility that the sexes might respond differently to the teaching and to the structural features of the school organization, nor has much consideration been given to the nature of the beliefs and values that students are expected to assimilate and the extent to which these are male beliefs and values. In her book on women doctors, Judith Lorber says (Lorber, 1984):

> my recollection was that there had been no women subject in *Boys in White*, *The Student Physician*, or any major study of physicians. My own review of these works confirmed my initial reaction – the

major studies of medical education in the United States were all on men, as was the classic analysis of physician's career development through patronage and sponsorship.

This situation applied in Britain as well, and only in recent years have some studies of women students begun to appear.

What are the values, beliefs and expectations that students must acquire while they practise 'how to play doctor'? What are the rules? They are not, of course, written down; there exists no moral code book which can be memorized. As with socialization for other adult roles, students slowly come to grips with the requirements of their putative profession and it is no easy task for researchers to spell out just what these requirements are. There are, however, a number of general observations that sociologists have put forward regarding medical values.

One such observation has to do with the paths by which students get to medical school. In the United States, as in Canada, Britain and Australia, the extremely competitive nature of admission is apparent. Medical schools have a wide choice among pupils coming up from lower schools and they choose the highest achievers, sometimes admitting them without interview. Where interviews are conducted, selection committees often feel uneasy about relying on the impressions gained therefrom and fall back on grades and scores (Mumford, 1983, p. 308). The subjects in which high achievements will count most for admission are likely to be in the sciences, chemistry, physics and biology being especially valued; this despite research indications that achievement in school science, as measured by scores and grades, is a notoriously bad predictor of clinical performance after graduation (Korman and Stubblefield 1971; Richards *et al.*, 1974; Burstein, 1981).

Thus, to students, the message appears to be that intense competitiveness and a scientific approach are prerequisites of progress in medical education. Emily Mumford (1983) however, points out that concentration on examination results reduces students' chances of taking part in pursuits which may contribute to their personal development and so to their future usefulness as physicians. Most of the people dealing with admissions are pursuing research and scientific work in academic environments and, themselves products of the system, are likely not to find much appeal in a student 'who is not academically brilliant or grade-motivated, even though such a person's patience and love of individual human beings might stand out like a beacon compared with some smooth-interview applicants'. She adds, 'it is easier to feel confidence in one's judgement about brilliance than in one's judgements about kindness, generosity, dependability and honesty' (p. 310).

During the years in medical school, an intellectual 'scientific' approach to medical practice, cool appraisal of problems, an impersonal stance and lack of emotional involvement with patients are much emphasized. It is also frequently stressed that practising medicine demands total dedication to work, an 'all-or-nothing' commitment, and the taking of 'responsibility' for clinical judgements and the lives of patients (Freidson, 1975a; Gordon, 1980).

Drawing on personal experience Gail Young describes the situation thus (Young, 1981, p. 146):

> The average student entering medical school will be primarily a scientist. The course in the first few years of medical school perpetuates this emphasis: the volume of work is increased so that there is an overwhelming amount of dry facts to be learned and teaching is mainly in groups of over a hundred in huge, impersonal lecture halls. The work seems to be only remotely related to looking after ill people. The whole approach to human beings is mechanistic, rationalist and analytical. Creativity and original thinking are easily quashed by the need to remember facts and regurgitate them for frequent exams.

In the jejune atmosphere of medical schools, decribed by Young, women students fare differently from their male counterparts. They are early made aware of a typecasting which assigns to them the 'human values' area of medical activity. Research evidence shows that it is the male students who are expected to shine in areas evaluated as crucial, e.g. a scientific approach to medicine, research, an unemotional stance and cool competence. Women are given the edge in patience, kindness and being good with people but these qualities are not highly rated. In an interesting study, Linda Grant explored peer expectations of medical students (Grant, 1983). She found that a student's gender had a systematic impact on evaluations of her or his competence by fellow students. In this research, students were asked to nominate fellows whom they thought most likely to achieve certain goals of medical knowledge and practice. The results showed ten dimensions (or goals) to be male dominated (i.e. most of those predicted to attain them were male), and among these were 'best knowledge of medical science', 'best researcher in medical science', 'most respected by professional peers', 'most competent clinician' and 'greatest contributor to medicine'. Only one dimension of medical competence was female dominated – 'sensitivity to patients' (Grant, 1983).

Grant argues that (p. 43)

> for most medical students, peer groups are critical support mechanisms and important arenas for professional socialization.

Not only do students spend a great deal of time with peers, but they also use them as 'social mirrors' to forge images of themselves as professionals.

Thus, peer evaluations can enforce values and expectations about the place of women in the medical profession. Grant's study reveals that female medical students are seen by their fellows as likely to shine in 'sensitivity to patients' (a quality habitually attributed to nurses) but likely to do less well in areas which, according to the value system of medical schools, constitute the essence of being a doctor.

During the socialization process in medical schools, female students are given to understand in ways both subtle and unsubtle that they are not expected to rise high in their chosen professional career. According to a number of U.S. studies, medical school staff, academic and administrative, hold that women students are less likely than their male equivalents to excel in scientific and research careers in medicine; they are not expected to become high-fliers (Bourne and Winkler, 1978; Scadron *et al.*, 1982). In such assessments the hierarchy of medical schools differs not at all from the peer attitudes reported by Grant. To the stereotyped view of women as being better suited to nurturing and caring roles, rather than scientific and diagnostic ones, is added the expectation that, like business women generally, female doctors will suffer from the career/family dichotomy. Such views and expectations are hard to change and those few women who have achieved eminence in their chosen spheres of activity tend to be dismissed as 'untypical'.

How do female medical students cope with the stresses stemming from low expectations and a typecasting which they resent? As said earlier, many feel that they have to try harder in order to show themselves to be the men's equal, and there is some support for the argument that this tendency to compete more and try harder increases during their years as students, possibly setting a pattern for future professional life. Spiegel *et al.* studied the relationship between stress, morale and academic performance in male and female medical students (Spiegel *et al.*, 1986) and came up with a quite striking pattern (p. 1161):

For women, the association between ratings of interpersonal stress and grades was found to be positive, suggesting that female medical students may react to conflicts in a way that enhances their academic performance. It has been reported that many female medical students and residents consider themselves challenged by male stereotypes of women and feel a need to prove their competence in this, as yet, male-dominated profession. If so, female students may be more likely than males to react to conflicts by increasing their effort and determination to succeed.

The authors of this paper (Spiegel *et al.*, 1986, p. 1161) continue by pointing out that

> it would be a mistake, however, to conclude from this that the stresses of medical education are benign or even healthy for women students. If women work harder than men to overcome the handicap of their minority status, it is clear that they do so at greater cost to their emotional and physical well-being.

Indeed, a number of researchers have concluded that female medical students suffer more from stress-related symptoms, and in general have more health problems, than do the men. Thus, for example, Grossman *et al.*, (1987), studying the coping resources and the health of male and female medical students, found that the women reported significantly more health problems than did the men. (The interpretation of such a finding is controversial, because women in general report more health problems than do men, a statistic that may reflect a greater willingness to report problems rather than a greater experience of them. However, the point made here is that trying ever harder to demonstrate that women are able to excel may well take its toll.)

Other researchers have made related findings: female medical students report more feelings of isolation and loneliness, greater difficulties in making new friends and, especially the married ones, a sense of being uncomfortable because they felt 'different' from their fellows (Hoferek and Sarnowski, 1981). Women students may need, and where possible have greater recourse to, the support of friends and families to combat such feelings of loneliness, etc. (Grossman *et al.*, 1987).

Male medical students, of course, also experience stresses, difficulties and unpleasant experiences during their years in medical school. Indeed, the argument is not at all that it is easy for them; studies have demonstrated their problems from the early work of Merton and Becker (Merton *et al.*, 1957; Becker *et al.*, 1961) to later findings that they turn to alcohol (more than women do) in order to cope with problems. The point is rather that female students receive a different kind of treatment, that they obtain less encouragement, and have to put up with a more damaging typecasting, than is the case with the male students.

Is it possible that women students themselves contribute to the stereotypical image and reduced expectations which they encounter, by entering medical schools predisposed to finding condescending attitudes and so starting with diminished confidence in their prospects? As already said, women are from infancy subject to a socialization which defines the roles seen as appropriate for them. There is some indication that female students tend to underrate their abilities and achievements, a usual tendency among women, and to attribute their attainments to a mixture of extraordinary effort and good luck (Grossman *et al.*, 1987). Grant, however, did not find any marked tendency among female medical students to denigrate or devalue either their own achievements and skills or those of fellow female students (Grant, 1983). All in all, it might be supposed that medical schools, like other institutions, do no more than reflect the gender structure of society and that the difficulties which confront the female student, and their responses, are an integral part of prevailing social mores. The atmosphere in medical schools might change in the final years of this century with the arrival of ever more female students but, to revert to Lorber (1984), evidence so far is to the contrary.

As is the case with medical-school students, those entering schools of nursing, physiotherapy, occupational therapy, etc., face ever more taxing courses as scientific knowledge expands and increasingly sophisticated equipment and appliances are made available. Furthermore, these students get caught up in the struggle to attain increasingly higher levels of achievement as their various occupational groups reach out for parity of esteem with the medical and other established professions.

Female students of these schools find themselves in a different kind of setting to that confronting medical-school entrants. For one thing, for the greater part of the present century, the majority of both teachers and students have been female and although this is slowly changing as more men enter these health occupations, women still constitute a numerical majority; the ambience is female, unlike the male-dominated medical schools. The other main difference, also changing even if more slowly, lies in the structure of the training programmes; traditionally entry requirements were less rigorous, the course shorter and career expectations lower than medical school equivalents. In Britain, during the 1980s, a small but growing number of students in nursing and the other health occupations attended courses which lead to university or equivalent degrees, with more such courses planned for the next two decades. In the United States, 'college-trained' nurses have been part of the health scene for very much longer.

Because female students in many health occupations form a majority, it is tempting and easy to assume that their situation is quite different from, and better than, that of women medical students. Certainly, there are differences: they do not have to struggle to prove themselves the equals of their male fellows and they may reasonably expect to rise high in their own hierarchies. (This latter may change in response to the male challenge, an issue which will be discussed later.) Many of the highest positions in the occupational hierarchies have been filled by women; for example, the stereotype boss of nurses is the 'matron'. It is likely then, that feelings of isolation and loneliness, experienced by women medical students as a result of perceived low status, are not the lot of women students elsewhere.

However, there are considerable shared experiences in the lives of women students, whether training to be doctors, midwives, physiotherapists or other health workers. They share the early experiences of girls in society, the usual socialization for gender stereotypes during childhood. Indeed, it is quite surprising to listen to students in the various health occupations still assuming that the medical profession is all 'male', seemingly unaware of the increasing numbers of women medical students. For example, the author, recently attending a seminar session of a group of occupational therapy students, 80 per cent of whom were female, was astonished to hear that they were expecting eventually to work with male doctors only; even when challenged they stuck to the view that the number of women doctors they would encounter would be 'negligible'. The stereotype 'doctor equals male' was marked.

Among girls of school age, the cultural expectation is that whatever their training, they will get married, have children and become immersed in family life. Studies show that the majority of female students in the health occupations adhere to the same expectation, and scant attention has so far been paid to the ways in which the domestic scene and the issue of women's work and roles has been presented to these students. Certainly these topics are included in most social science courses, which form part of the curriculum in nursing and occupational therapy, and increasingly figure in the programmes of medical schools and physiotherapy schools. These topics are central to the preparation of health visitors, social workers and others whose duties take them among families. It is a matter of regret, therefore, that the social sciences as taught to students of these subjects in universities and colleges, are all too often based on male theoretical views with hardly more than a nod, if that, towards feminist thinking. A recent survey of the books and articles prescribed for use in social science courses for occupational therapists and physiotherapists revealed an absence of works by feminist writers. The very considerable scholarship, the insights and the research contributions made by these writers to sociology and psychology, were totally ignored. This state of affairs is deplorable – firstly, because educational institutions are expected to present material in a way that is both balanced and objective, giving weight to all sides of an argument. Ignoring the feminist contribution distorts and misleads. Secondly, many of the students will eventually find themselves working with women, sometimes as colleagues, frequently as clients and patients. If they are indoctrinated only with the male view of women they will practise according to this view and so perpetuate it.

Jean Orr (Orr, 1986, p. 75) says that

> A study of student health visitors' perception of women showed the extent to which they were influenced by sex-role stereotyping. Women were seen as passive, dependent, sentimental and afraid of change, with little control over many aspects of their lives. Women were said to have characteristics of warmth and express-iveness, while men were said to have characteristics in the com-petence realm.
>
> Essentially health visitor students have a patriarchal view of the world, and there is little evidence of any other perspective being presented during the course. What they receive is a male view of the world, masquerading as science.

This kind of teaching is very likely to influence the work of future generations of health workers. It is a curious feature of education in many health-related courses that while women in general are charac-terized as emotional, expressive and submissive, the (mostly female) students themselves are taught to adhere to the supposed male virtues, or neutrality, lack of emotion and cool-headedness. The possibility that this may engender conflict in female students is apparently ignored. For example Jane Salvage says of nurse-training, 'Nurses are not sup-posed to show their feelings; crying when a patient dies is getting 'too' involved and is frowned on as unprofessional' (Salvage, 1985).

The female student, being prepared for a career in one of the health occupations, will thus find, in her university or college training, a continuance of the sex-stereotyping previously encountered. When she moves out of the lecture hall to receive practical instruction in a hospital, health centre or other health setting, she will find herself confronted by the realities of the gender division of labour in the health-care business. She will observe the (male) doctors at the top of the hierarchy with her own occupational group accorded an inferior position. She will realize, also, her own low ranking within that group. Coming to terms with this situation, which may well influence her future work with colleagues and patients, can be painful.

One student nurse, quoted by Salvage (1985, p. 89), describes

> the attitude of deference to medical staff and to all senior nursing staff. This deference goes beyond what is called for by the system of line management ... this habitual deference may largely be responsible for nurses' reluctance to speak out for what we feel is right or needs changing. We are often afraid to take a stand against those above us in the hierarchy.

Working in a male-dominated profession: women doctors

With the increase in the number of women graduating from medical schools, the proportion of women medical practitioners is rising. Table 5.1 shows this profession over a 10-year period, 1976 to 1986, during which the number of female hospital medical staff in England grew from 18.6 per cent to 24.8 per cent of the total. During a comparable period, 1975 to 1985, the proportion of women principals in general practice ('unrestricted principals') in England increased from 12.9 per cent to 19.0 per cent (DHSS, 1986).

Thus, despite a lessening of the imbalance that leaves women doctors in a minority of the profession, their situation continues to be more like that of women in other male-dominated professions such as law, civil service and university teaching than of women in the other health occupations. For example, in England & Wales the proportion of women lawyers (solicitors) was 12.3 per cent in 1984 (Spencer and Podmore, 1987); in UK universities, women academics form under 10 per cent of the total and the figure for the higher Civil Service is much the same. When considering the characteristics of the work setting and the experiences of women doctors it is of interest to draw on research findings relating to women's work in other 'male' professions. Studies such as that by Spencer and Podmore (1987) on women lawyers, by Walters (1987) on women in the Civil Service, and by Newton (1987) on female engineers all demonstrate the same pattern: in these professions, the higher the grade or status, the lower the proportion of women among them.

Table 5.2 shows how this pattern also applies to hospital doctors. In England & Wales, in 1986, the proportion of female house officers was almost 40 per cent; of consultants less than 14 per cent. When it comes to promotion, the dice are loaded in favour of male doctors.

Women doctors, then, are not equally distributed among the various hospital grades; neither are they equally distributed among the various

Table 5.1 Hospital medical staff in England

Sex	1976	1983	1986
Male	29 815	33 077	33 101
Female	6 798	9 632	10 891
Total	36 613	42 709	43 992

Source: Manpower Statistics, 1986.

Table 5.2 Hospital medical staff by grade and sex in England in 1986

Staff	Male	Female	Total
Consultants	11 913	1 872	13 785
Senior Registrars	2 443	810	3 253
Registrar	4 497	1 352	5 849
Senior House Officer	6 437	3 253	9 690
House Officer	1 614	1 191	2 813

Source: *Manpower Statistics*, 1987.

medical specialties. More are to be found in community medicine, school medicine, geriatric medicine, anaesthetics, mental handicap and (especially in the United States) paediatrics; far fewer are in most branches of surgery, obstetrics and internal medicine. This is a significant feature of the situation of women doctors and suggests that they are, in fact, 'marginalized'. According to Heins and Braslow (1981), a similar situation prevails in many Western countries.

How does this situation come about? There is considerable evidence of a marked difference between male and female doctors with regard to the factors influencing career decisions (Hutt, 1981). These factors affect not only initial choices, made after graduation, but they affect subsequent decisions, taken during early or mid-career, as to whether to stay with the first choice or try some other specialty. What are these factors?

Broadly, three factors can be cited as strongly influencing women's career choices in medicine: (1) their greater acceptance in specialties which appear to value aptitudes stereotyped as natural attributes of women, e.g. interpersonal skills, sensitivity and patience; (2) the attraction of specialties in which the conflict between family commitment and work responsibilities can be minimized; and (3) lesser competition from men in specialties which carry lower pay and prestige, thus making entry for women easier.

A number of researchers have studied the mechanics of entry into the various medical specialties. As mentioned earlier, women medical students are often seen, and some see themselves, as being especially suited to work where the stereotypical 'nurturing' skills of women can be utilized (Grant, 1983). Also, there are preconceived notions of the characteristics and skills required for particular medical specialties: for example, surgeons are expected to be unemotional, cool and detached from their patients while paediatricians should be involved and emotionally sensitive (Lorber, 1984, p. 32), two contrasting notions which together produce a dilemma typical of those which can confront women striving to make headway in male-dominated professions. Thus, Spencer and Podmore (Spencer and Podmore, 1987, p. 2), in their study of lawyers, found that there were, on the one hand

stereotypes about women – for example that women's innate characteristics mean that they are 'emotional', 'unstable', 'not decisive enough'

and on the other hand there were

stereotypes about the nature of professions and professionals – for example that professions are 'physically demanding', 'combative' and hence unsuited to women.

The real personalities and skills of women doctors may not match their stereotypes, any more than the actual job demands fit the preconceived requirements, but popular impressions exert a powerful influence both in the shaping of specialty choices and in career advice. There has been little research into this contrast between the perceived skills requirements of specialties, and the true needs thereof, but what there is indicates the possibility that stereotyped expectations are not borne out by reality. Cartwright and Anderson (1981) in their study of general practitioners, showed that although the expectation may be that women are more caring and sensitive to patients, the reality is of a marked similarity between male and female general practitioners in such (and other) respects. Nevertheless, female GPs are often steered towards particularly 'feminine' tasks.

Stereotyping, then, is one major factor influencing the career choices of women doctors. Another is their expectation that eventual marriage and child-bearing would conflict with work responsibilities and that this conflict would be more pronounced in some fields than in others. Not only does this potential conflict affect initial choices, the actual experience of it can result in a career-switch, a transfer to fields where the problem can be minimized.

The majority of women doctors are married and a substantial proportion of them are married to doctors. In a survey of two cohorts of women graduating from UK medical schools, Audrey Ward found that 83 per cent of an early cohort and 89 per cent of a late cohort were married (Ward, 1982). Over half (55 per cent) of these married doctors' husbands were themselves doctors or dentists. (It is of interest to note that 76 per cent of all husbands were in social class I.) Other studies showed quite similar results. Stephen (1987), for example, found that 10 years after graduation from UK medical schools, 18 per cent of women were single and that 47 per cent of the married graduates had married doctors.

Several studies have demonstrated that married women's choice of medical specialty, and of situation applied for, are much influenced by domestic considerations. The majority of married women doctors, according to Stephen's study, have at least one child (Stephen, 1987). As a consequence, the female doctor frequently seeks a part-time post, or one which offers flexible working hours, besides which its location needs to be within easy reach of home; many change their jobs to fit in with the employment movements of their husbands. Audrey Ward found that about half (49 per cent) of the married women doctors in her sample considered that domestic commitments, the family's need for their care, had affected the choice of jobs they felt in a position to apply for, and almost as many (41 per cent) thought they had been restricted in job applications by their husbands' career requirements (Ward, 1982). Rosemary Hutt and her colleagues (1981) found, in their manpower studies of doctors, that women doctors had opted to work in the specialties in which they were engaged at the time of the study, at a later stage in their careers than had the men. This may reflect career changes due to a family move or to having children. Far more women than men, in this study, said that geographical location had been a factor of great importance in their specialty decision; working hours and fitting in with family circumstances were other important factors. Indeed, nearly half of the women said that the availability of a part-time post had been of great importance in their decision. On the other hand, many fewer women than men had been influenced in career choices by considerations of better pay, good prospects and good equipment.

This pattern of choosing employment strongly resembles that of married women possessed of little by way of training or qualifications. Mothers of young children, especially, frequently seek 'convenient' work, which fits in with domestic duties, at the expense of accepting lower pay, inferior status and absence of job security (Sharpe, 1984; Miles, 1988).

In the medical profession, the fields of, for example, anaesthetics, school medicine and community medicine, offer opportunities for part-time employment and are therefore popular with married women doctors. In these specialties it is relatively easy to organize work on a sessional basis. The drawback of such employment is that it usually offers less attractive career prospects, lower status, fewer opportunities to attain higher qualifications and to do research, than does full-time work. It also contradicts a prevailing medical value, the 'all-or-nothing', total commitment to work; therefore it is viewed with suspicion (*British Medical Journal*, 1980).

Anaesthetics does involve high technology which would make it attractive to male doctors. The problem possibly is that it is a sort of dead-end specialty – the surgeon does the prestige work.

The third factor which influences women doctors' career choices is the relative unpopularity of certain specialties with doctors. Such may carry low status, new technological medicine may be inappropriate and 'miracle' cures are unlikely. Mental handicap, geriatric medicine, and the care of many chronic conditions fall into this category of unpopular specialties which therefore attract fewer doctors and in which the competition for places is less fierce than elsewhere. Female students and junior doctors may be attracted to these fields precisely because the chances of entry, and of subsequent advancement, seem better than in those specialties towards which the ambitious male doctors gravitate. They may also find themselves subtly channelled into the less popular specialties (a) because the male doctors do not compete for them, and (b) by subtle emphasis on the particular suitability of women in caring for patients who may be thought unlikely to benefit from any treatment other than routine medication and for whom the 'womanly' qualities of kindness and patience may be of equal or more importance.

The features of specialty choices in medicine so far discussed, stereotyping, the dichotomy of work and family, and the comparatively better opportunities in unpopular jobs, combine to marginalize women doctors, i.e. keep them away from the prestigious core, or mainstream, of the medical profession. As said earlier, their situation is not dissimilar to that of women in other male-dominated professions; for example, Spencer and Podmore (1987, p. 113) note that women lawyers

> find that they are not very welcome and that the ways in which they can use their knowledge and abilities are controlled and channelled by a variety of mechanisms, often insidious. For example certain areas of work will be relatively inaccessible to them: other areas will be foisted upon them as 'appropriate' to women.

Lorber (1984) suggests that for women the rationale of choosing a medical specialty is to feel welcome and comfortable in it and that this is more likely to be the case in areas where women are already accepted. Unfortunately, any such tendency serves to reinforce the stereotyping of women and of certain specialties as being 'women's province'.

For women to feel unwelcome, inferior and marginalized in their workplace can happen in most fields of medicine even in general practice where, although in a minority (under 20 per cent in Britain) women appear to be accepted (Eisner and Wright, 1986). In general practice the interpersonal skills, patience and caring, which are seen as feminine skills, are regarded as valuable to doctors (Young, 1981, p. 155). Nevertheless, it is frequently the case that women GPs are channelled into dealing with particular types of problems or patients.

Lawrence (Lawrence, 1987, p. 152) called this 'ghettoism', a strong word, by which she means a situation

> when women doctors find themselves seeing specific categories of patients in a group practice – many of the women, especially for specifically 'women's problems' (gynaecological, obstetrics and family planning), many of the psychiatric cases (a large proportion of whom are women), and the paediatric cases, especially when children are brought along to the surgery by mothers.

The implication here is that this kind of specialization within a medical specialty is not sought by the women doctors but is imposed on them. Lawrence argues that women doctors frequently choose general practice because it appears to offer a wide range of medical experience and they do not wish to have themselves limited to particular work within it. In her study of single-handed women GPs, this imposed ghettoism was mentioned by several female doctors as a snag in working within group practices, and as a reason for leaving them. She quoted examples (Lawrence, 1987, p. 152), such as:

> In the practice that we joined, there were four men so . . . I was doing mainly gynae and maternity and paediatrics and seeing children.
> We had got the midwife to give a little bit of help in ante-natal but I was doing the whole lot.

Of course there is nothing wrong about women doctors specializing in women's problems – on the contrary, there appears to be a very real demand for this from patients; it is its imposition by male colleagues on unwilling women doctors that rankles. Other women general practitioners mentioned their exclusion from decision-making, especially when they work part-time, and the allocation of women and child patients to them as 'lady doctors' in partnerships, as ways of making them less than equal (Eisner and Wright, 1986).

Many writers, discussing the problems of women in largely male professions mention the 'double-bind' in which such women find themselves. Double-bind is a situation when contradictory demands are placed on a person, so that whatever action is taken, this appears to be wrong. The classic double-bind for professional women is that conforming to a profession's male values, behaving like men in their professional roles, and competing with men as men compete with each other, lays them open to the criticism of being unfeminine, while to work differently from male colleagues and not always conform to male values exposes them to the accusation of being unprofessional, even incompetent. A woman doctor is seen, and is expected to be, warm, sensitive, and understanding in a culture where emotional detachment, objectivity and coolness are valued. In this situation she tries either to become an acceptable and valued professional, albeit unfeminine and unnatural, or a 'feminine', and thus devalued one. The expectations are incompatible.

Little attention has been paid by researchers to the differential experiences of single and married women doctors, perhaps because most women doctors are married. It is possible, however, that single women are accepted more into the male culture of the medical profession than are married women, especially mothers of young children.

Female doctors are not the only women who work in health occupations dominated by men. Female dentists, pharmacists, scientific and technical staff in hospital laboratories, share many of the problems faced by women doctors. A study of women scientists in the British National Health Service, by Hilary Homans (1987), is especially interesting because it throws some light on how male colleagues and hospital managers see female scientists (graduate biochemists and others). Homans (p. 91) found a strong tendency in male managers to assume that women scientists would leave the service on pregnancy and not return, thus being a liability causing high turnover rates:

> This study found clear evidence that selection and promotion practices are based on certain myths about women, the most pervasive myths being that all women will leave to have babies and that wastage due to pregnancy is greater than for any other reason.

In fact when she examined data on wastage rates, Homans found that not all women left to have children, many wished to return after maternity leave, and that much wastage was due to men leaving the NHS to go to jobs in industry with better payment and career prospects. Certainly pregnancy was not the largest cause of wastage. Male managers in this study, however, often expressed the view that women with children should not work. Like women doctors, women scientists find themselves pushed into less prestigious, less desirable work, which is regarded as more 'suitable' for women: Homans found 'statistically significant evidence that men spent more time than women on research, staff management and administration' (p. 103), tasks likely to lead to promotion. Women scientists, like their medical colleagues, have to prove their dedication by showing that they do not intend to have children and are completely committed to their careers.

Working in a 'female profession'

It could be expected that compared to working in a male-dominated occupation, women who work in a predominantly female profession

Table 5.3 Nursing staff in hospitals and at district

Nursing staff	1975	1985
Whole-time male	33 240	38 668
Whole-time female	164 484	211 586
Part-time male	2 948	1 697
Part-time female	131 522	131 995
Total	332 194	383 946

Source: Manpower Statistics, 1987.

would find their situation relatively problem-free. The reality is different, and curiously, women in, for example, nursing, occupational therapy and physiotherapy, occupations where the majority of the employees are women, experience problems very similar to those faced by female doctors and scientists. As Table 5.3 shows, the majority of nurses are female, and a considerable number of them work part time. Only a little over 10 per cent of all nurses are males and of these only a small proportion work part time.

Despite its being a traditionally female occupation (indeed the nurse is stereotyped in society as female) promotion for women in nursing is not straightforward: the higher the grade and status, the more men are to be found there. This is also true of other 'female occupations' such as occupational therapy or physiotherapy. What is more, the situation is not improving. Indeed, writing about nurses in Britain, Trevor Clay (1987, p. 111) argued that

> the introduction of general management, which has dislodged and in many places destroyed the nursing hierarchies, has knocked many female nursing managers out of the scene and created an NHS management with an overwhelming male ethos.

Clay quoted figures which showed that in 1983 almost 44 per cent of District Nursing Officers were men and that men formed a high proportion of nursing general managers in the mid-1980s. Thus, even in female professions, men have better chances of promotion than do women.

The reasons are similar to those prevailing in medicine, which is hardly surprising, given that all occupational groups function within the power structure of the larger society. Female nurses, like women doctors, marry and bear children. They want their work to fit in with their domestic and child-care arrangements and for many, this inevitably means part-time work. Part-time employment is certainly available for nurses (see Table 5.3) but, as elsewhere, promotion prospects are good only for full-timers. In this context, it is interesting to note that many nurses who have left, or are seriously thinking of leaving nursing, often say that the provision of crèche and child-care facilities would attract them back, or encourage them to stay (Clay, 1987). Full-time nursing, with enhanced career prospects, would become a possibility for many such women if suitable arrangements for their children were made available but this is a common need throughout industry and commerce also and one that is only slowly and tentatively being met.

There are other problems which confront mothers in nursing. Pregnant women find it difficult to carry out some nursing duties, especially as pregnancy advances, and nursing uniforms cannot accommodate pregnancy. Taking a long break from nursing brings questions of continued competence. While shift-work may seem to be a feature of nursing which is helpful to women with young children, this is not necessarily the case. Night shifts, long shifts, and the system of internal rotation, are bearable for women without children but intolerable for nurse-mothers.

However, the difficulties faced by women in nursing go deeper than mere work arrangements. Some of the underlying attitudes in nursing are similar to those found in medical practice. An all-or-nothing commitment to the profession is often demanded of nurses, and this, almost by definition, cannot be given by women with children. The model for such commitment, and consequent advancement, might have been designed to give men and single women a head start. Not surprisingly, observers of the nursing profession question the necessity, even the usefulness, of this all-or-nothing commitment (Oakley, 1984b) and emphasize the excellent contribution that nurses who are also mothers can make.

It may also be argued that the requirement of 'obedience', painfully learnt during socialization into nursing, is harmful not only to the overall status of nursing, but to the advancement of women within it. The occupation of nursing is strictly hierarchical and authoritarian, run on a military model, where a clear allocation of tasks and responsibility for control is held to be of extreme importance. In such a structure, unquestioning obedience to those in more senior positions is seen as essential. Obedience, not only to doctors, but to senior nursing staff is demanded of nurses. Indeed, various writers on features of contemporary nursing have commented on the painful process of learning to be a nurse and on the self-perpetuating system of demanding obedience. Jane Salvage writes (Salvage, 1985):

Many senior nurses behave in such a heartless and insulting way to juniors that it is hard to believe they have been through similar experiences themselves. But therein perhaps lies the key; the experience of becoming a nurse and rising through the ranks leaves so many scars that self-protection is the only route most people can follow. Insecurity, lack of confidence, lack of assertiveness and the often unrealistic expectations of other people may provoke a very natural human response of defensiveness, so that at least on the surface one can appear indestructible.

It is indeed likely that diffidence and unassertiveness, typical of women in general, are characteristic of nurses also, especially those who are married, with children, and so have small prospects of advancement in their chosen career. As in other areas of employment, women back down in the face of male competition and male power in nursing, because they lack confidence. In Ann Oakley's words (Oakley, 1984):

If Florence Nightingale had trained her lady pupils in assertiveness rather than obedience, perhaps nurses would be in a different place now.

6

Patients and professionals: patterns of interaction

Relationships between patients and health professionals

A consultation between a health professional (doctor, nurse or other therapist) and a patient, is a 'social' encounter: the two participants come to the consultation each with a set of expectations as to how they will both behave and each with one or more goals which they want to attain. Actual behaviour during the consultation is influenced by the expectations and goals of the two participants and by the perception by each of the conduct of the other. Whether expectations are shared or different, whether the goals are similar or not, will have a major impact on the consultation.

Patients' relationships with doctors have been much researched: the nature of consultations; patterns of communication, diversity of goals and consequent bargaining during consultations, sources of satisfaction and dissatisfaction with the consultation process, all have received attention (see, for example, Cartwright, 1967; Stimson and Webb, 1975; Byrne and Long, 1976; Tuckett et al., 1985). By comparison, similar aspects of patients' relationships with professionals other than doctors have been less studied so that discussion of research findings tends to focus mostly on patients' encounters with doctors. Indeed, doctors, as the most powerful profession in the health labour force, have been able to influence the expectations, the goals and the actions of patients and of other professionals, dominating the consultation process to an extent that these others have not matched, a factor which may explain research bias towards the study of patients' relationships with doctors rather than with these other professionals.

In earlier studies of doctor–patient relationships, the gender of the two participants was virtually ignored. The assumption, usually unstated, appeared to be that the gender of doctor and patient did not influence interaction between them. In that, researchers may have accepted the convention of the western medical profession that doctors are somewhat 'sexless' and 'genderless' beings, and therefore that patients could talk to them, undress in front of them and be examined by them in an 'asexual' way. Little attempt was made to discover whether patients in reality perceived doctors in this way. Another convention of Western medical practice, that doctors treat all patients alike, regardless of gender, or indeed of class or other attributes, was also largely unquestioned. Thus, it was sociological work concerned with social class and health care which first began to raise the issue of the expectations and actions of doctors and patients being influenced by gender and by their class background (see, for example, Cartwright and O'Brien, 1976).

More recent studies have looked at the effect of gender on interaction between patients and doctors and have sought to find answers to such questions as whether doctors relate to and treat their female and male patients differently, whether women patients prefer to be treated by male or female doctors, whether there are systematic variations in patterns of relationships according to the gender of doctor and patient, and whether such issues are likely to affect medical care.

Female and male doctors: differences in attitudes

A growing volume of literature indicates that while doctors may subscribe to the ethical requirement of not differentiating between patients on the basis of class, race, gender, or past behaviour, they do not, in reality, think about or treat their patients in an objective, uniform way. Several researchers have noted that doctors categorize patients as 'good' and 'bad', or as 'problem' or 'easy' patients. For example, Lorber (1975) found that doctors regard as 'good' those hospital patients who do not make trouble, or complain or interrupt medical routines. Stimson (1976) noted the willingness of British general practitioners to categorize their patients: in a postal questionnaire, answered by 453 doctors (gender undistinguished), Stimson asked doctors to give a sketch of patients who 'caused the least trouble' and 'the most trouble'. Doctors did not refuse to answer, as might have been expected, on the basis of ethical prescriptions such as 'all patients are the same' or 'no patient is too much trouble'. On the contrary, doctors found it possible to answer and only 7 per cent of those who returned the questionnaire did not complete this section. The results showed that women patients were widely held to be 'more trouble' than the men and that patients presenting the doctor with organic, physical and treatable diseases were considered less trouble than those who complained of emotional and psychiatric problems (mainly women) and those with chronic diseases.

Not only do doctors categorize patients (as good or bad) according to how much trouble they cause to them in their work, they also make normative judgements of their patients and think of them as good or bad individuals, for example as good wife, bad employee, bad mother or good son. These judgements are not made according to any medical criteria, but according to the doctors' personal, culturally determined value as to what a mother, employee or son should be.

In her study *Single and Pregnant*, Sally Macintyre (1977a) showed that consultations for unwanted pregnancies triggered categorizations of women by doctors as 'good' or 'bad'. The 'bad girl' was one who was promiscuous, 'easy-going', 'immoral' according to the values of the doctor, and who was seen to have become pregnant as a result of bad behaviour. 'Good girl' was applied to one seen by the doctor as 'innocent', who became pregnant because someone had 'taken advantage' of her. Similar categorization based on personal value judgements was found by a study conducted in the southern United States by Fisher and Groce (1985). They gathered information from a teaching hospital's family practice clinic, where 43 medical interviews with women patients were audio and video-taped. The women were all new patients and doctors evaluated them as good or bad women during the interviews, according to their own cultural assumptions.

In most research of this kind, the doctors studied were male and few investigators explored whether female doctors categorized their patients in similar ways. It is likely, however, that female doctors have different values and therefore see their women patients' roles in a different light from their male colleagues. It can be argued that women doctors are likely to have different political and ideological views than male doctors concerning the position of women in society not only because they share the socialization and other experiences of women in general, but also because they themselves have broken out of the traditional pattern of women's lives by becoming doctors. Their assumptions about women's place and roles and about the nature of women are thus likely to differ markedly from those of male doctors, an argument confirmed by studies in the United States and Canada where it was found by Heins *et al.* (1979) in Detroit, and by Leichner and Harper (1982) in Canada, that female doctors are more likely to be aware of gender issues, and to be sympathetic to feminist views of women than are male doctors. Others noted that female medical students are more sensitive to gender discrimination against both female doctors and patients (Leserman, 1981) and that female gynaecologists are more sympathetic to the feminist position on family size and women's roles than are their male counterparts (Margolis *et al.*, 1983).

Doctors' values and views are of the utmost importance to patients because they influence medical practice. Repeated findings demonstrate that the treatment accorded to patients may vary according to the cultural views and values held by their doctors. Thus, Sally Macintyre (1977a) found that doctors, having categorized women who consulted them with unwanted pregnancies as 'good girls' or 'bad girls', discriminated in their willingness to terminate the pregnancy according to such judgements. Her research demonstrated that differential medical management of problems can result from cultural judgements. Fisher and Groce (1985) neatly illustrated cases of differential treatment as between one woman and another, both treated by the same doctor. Maria, a 24-year-old, unmarried, Mexican–American patient, came to a clinic ostensibly with a leg injury following a motorbike accident, but also with an almost hidden agenda: she wanted to make enquiries about contraception and the possibilities of abortion, if needed. During the medical interview, the doctor formed an opinion of her as a women whose morals were at odds with the cultural norms of people in the conservative 'Bible-belt' country in which the clinic was located and where most doctors disapproved of abortion. Maria had already had several abortions and miscarriages, was sexually active but not practising birth control, and seemed in general a hard-drinking, promiscuous woman. At the end of the consultation, Maria left the clinic without the birth control advice she asked for, without information about abortion, without pain-killers or other medication for her presenting leg pain, and was discouraged from returning to the clinic. By contrast, another patient, Sarah, aged 23, from a conventional background, who appeared shy and well-behaved, who was also a sexually active unmarried woman, but did not seem promiscuous, having one boyfriend whom she planned to marry, was judged during the medical interview to be 'good' and reliable. Sarah left the clinic with advice on contraception, with all her problems dealt with and encouragement to return. Cultural judgements in these cases resulted in different treatment.

It is likely that women doctors with values more sympathetic to women who reject the traditional constraints of pregnancies and child-rearing, would treat women patients differently than did the male doctors referred to in the study of Fisher and Groce. Indeed, Margolis found that female gynaecologists were more likely to be sympathetic to women who wanted birth control advice to limit their family size and to women who requested abortions on grounds of already large families (Margolis *et al.*, 1983).

Female and male doctors: differences in interacting with patients

There may well be differences, in their modes of relating to patients, between female and male doctors because their essential experiences, their relative positions in the social structure and thus, their attitudes are gender-related.

There is some evidence that female doctors may be more willing than male doctors to form egalitarian relationships with patients. Traditionally, the largely male profession of medicine expected its patients to be deferential and submissive in interaction. It can be argued that female doctors, who as women are not used to playing dominant roles or expecting others to be submissive, are more willing to see patients as equal partners in consultations and readier to allow patients to make decisions. Especially when dealing with female patients, women doctors may be less likely than male doctors to assume that women are passive by nature, and that they need decisions to be made for them. There is insufficient research evidence to show the extent to which women doctors practise 'egalitarian' medicine; indeed, some women practitioners may wish to appear so 'male-like' in order to succeed in their careers that they are less rather than more egalitarian with patients. However, the study by Leichner and Harper (1982) indicated that women doctors generally are more likely to accept patients as equals.

Evidence has been adduced to show that female doctors spend more time with patients than do male doctors. Thus Langwell (1982) found that in the United States, in all specialties, female physicians saw fewer patients per hour and spent more time with each than did male physicians. The difference was most marked in gynaecology and obstetrics where male doctors saw almost twice the number of patients per hour as did female doctors. Similar were the findings of Cypress (1984) who studied the National Ambulatory Medical Care Survey in the United States and found that female physicians and female gynaecologists and obstetricians, in comparison to their male counterparts, spent on average more time in face-to-face contact with patients.

One explanation of this difference is that women doctors are more interested in talking with patients and the greater length of consultation reflects their interests and preferred working habits.

Another explanation is that women doctors are more skilful in communicating with patients and in developing rapport (Preston-Whyte *et*

al., 1983). Indeed, women are socialized into becoming more expressive, and more adept at explaining issues to others than are men whose
socialization inclines them to reticence. Consequently, women doctors
are likely to be better able to listen and to elicit information, and
patients in turn to find themselves more able to expand on their
problems, thus lengthening the time of consultation (Leserman, 1981).

American researchers also raised the possibility that women doctors,
being less well equipped and less senior than their male counterparts,
have fewer back-up staff (i.e. secretaries, records-clerks, etc.), an
added reason for more time being spent on each consultation.

Of course, more time spent with patients, by itself, does not necessarily lead to a better quality of medical care; much depends on how
the time is spent. Nevertheless, most studies of patients' preferences
show that people like longer consultations and think that they benefit
more from doctors who are willing to listen and to discuss their
problems.

Another indication that female doctors may interact differently with
their patients comes from a British study which showed that female
doctors had a significantly higher level of doctor-initiated appointments (Preston-Whyte *et al.*, 1983). The majority of such consultations
are 'follow-up' appointments, i.e. the patient is asked to return at a
given time. In the general practice where the study was conducted
female doctors had considerably higher follow-up rates, especially for
female patients with sex-specific problems. There could be an element
of 'one woman to another' in this, the researchers suggesting that
female doctors may also be more skilled in establishing rapport and
ensuring that patients do return, as asked.

Do doctors treat female and male patients differently?

As discussed, doctors, of both sexes, employ their personal values and
views of the world in categorizing their patients and the question arises
as to whether systematic differences are to be found in doctors'
methods of treating patients, according to the gender thereof. Treatment for the psychological problems of female patients has been much
debated, the argument going that doctors are inclined to regard a
variety of complaints made by women as emotional or psychological in
origin, not to be taken too seriously, while similar complaints from
men are given greater weight and are more thoroughly investigated.
Central to this argument is the stereotypical view, widely held in
Western society, of women as weak and unstable, given to complaining and exaggerating their discomforts. This view is prevalent among
men and accepted by many women and it would be surprising if

doctors (mostly male) did not share the views of the society of which they are a part (Leeson and Gray, 1978). If doctors think that women patients tend to maximize their discomfort and complain unduly, they may dismiss their problems lightly, thus providing inferior medical care.

This issue is contentious and difficult to resolve, partly because the evidence is contradictory and partly because the implications are unclear. In an influential study, Lennane and Lennane (1973), noted that doctors systematically dismissed or minimized certain female complaints. They were able to show that when women complained of severe pains during menstruation, of nausea and other symptoms in pregnancy and of unusually severe pain in childbirth, doctors often attributed these complaints to emotional or 'psychogenic' causes in the women concerned. The researchers argued that in spite of strong evidence of an organic basis of the complaints, the doctors regarded the women as having psychological problems and overstating the pain. The Lennanes were of the opinion that this treatment indicated a deeply rooted sex bias on the part of the doctors, who did not take women's pains seriously, and did not adequately investigate their causes.

Differential treatment given to male and female patients for similar complaints was noted by Bernstein and Kane (1981). They studied the attitudes of physicians towards female and male patients by using simulated cases (vignettes of patients' complaints and ways of presenting their problems to the doctor). The results showed that doctors responded differently to female and male patients, as depicted, some 25 per cent thinking that women were likely to make excessive demands on the time of physicians. Women's complaints were judged more likely to be influenced by emotional factors and were identified as psychosomatic more frequently than were men's complaints of a similar nature. Bernstein and Kane detected no difference as between male and female doctors, but very few of the doctors were female (225 male, and 28 female, doctors participated in the study).

Not only this study, and some others based on simulated cases, but some of those in which researchers were able to record real consultations, confirmed the case for differential treatment. Thus, Wallen *et al.* (1979) tape-recorded 336 consultations between U.S. male doctors and their patients, their analysis showing that these doctors were more likely to attribute psychological causes to the illnesses of female than of male patients, and so were more pessimistic in their prognoses: they regarded female patients as emotionally unstable and difficult to treat. Armitage *et al.* (1979) found that U.S. male patients received more services for comparable conditions.

The above-quoted researchers put one side of the argument, but other evidence suggests that the reality is more complex. Also using the simulation technique, McCranie *et al.* (1978) observed no gender bias. These researchers presented doctors with vignettes of patients complaining of chronic headaches or chronic abdominal pain, accompanied by some usual additional symptoms (these cases being selected because they could be indicative of either psychological or organic illness) and asked the doctors how they would handle these problems. The results of this study showed that while the doctors predominantly favoured organic explanations in making their initial diagnoses, they were not more inclined to diagnose women's symptoms as indicating psychological illness than they were those of men.

More influential have been the studies carried out by Lois Verbrugge and her colleagues who examined data from the National Ambulatory Medical Care Survey in the United States. They selected a number of common complaints (e.g. chest pain, back pain, headache, fatigue, dizziness) and studied the medical responses to patients who consulted doctors for these complaints (Verbrugge and Steiner, 1981). Their analysis revealed a systematic, but somewhat unexpected, difference in doctors' treatment of male and female patients: in about 30–40 per cent of the services and dispositions studied, gender differences occurred showing that women received more medical care. They noted that gender differences persisted even when patients' age, seriousness of problem and diagnosis were controlled. Women received more extensive services – more laboratory tests, blood-pressure checks, prescriptions and return appointments.

Not only are research results rather contradictory, but the interpretations that may be placed on gender-based differences in treatment are unclear. The core of the difficulty is that receiving increased medical attention may be seen as an advantage or as a disadvantage. On the one hand, it can be argued that it is in the patient's interest to receive a thorough medical investigation of problems, because such will lead to a better chance of treatment and cure, while dismissing complaints and neglecting to investigate them may well bring more pain and worse problems. On the other hand, more medical care for patients can be seen adversely: lives of patients may be 'over-medicalized', laboratory investigations may serve the doctors' interests as much, if not more, than those of the patients, and medical technology can be over-employed. Moreover, the use of medical intervention and technology is more easily effected on powerless, compliant sections of society such as female patients, and it has been suggested that intervention may be used as a form of punishment for complaining women.

Both interpretations have been put forward. Thus Lois Verbrugge argued that more tests and treatments are used on women who are easily intimidated and are seen as unduly complaining, while Armitage argued that doctors provide more treatment and care for men because they take their complaints more seriously and regard their return to work as more important.

It is also possible that the gender of the patient triggers a response in the doctor which results in a particular method of treatment. In this respect, differences in the prescribing of tranquillizers for women and for men has received much attention. It is certainly the case that female patients receive more prescriptions for tranquillizers than do male patients, but interpreting the prescribing habits of doctors is notoriously difficult. Ruth Copperstock and colleagues (1978, 1979) studied sex differences in the use of psychotropic drugs in Ontario, Canada. Her studies were based on computerized records of a prescription agency of prescriptions dispensed during certain time periods. She found that a consistently higher proportion of women than men received tranquillizers and that women went on using them for longer periods than did men. Cooperstock argued that this pattern was connected with doctors' differential perceptions of women and men, i.e. because women are expected to present them with many emotional and 'ill-defined' symptoms doctors prescribe tranquillizers for them more readily and without much thought as to alternatives.

Other studies showed similar patterns, for example, that amongst elderly institutionalized patients, women were given more tranquillizers than the men, even when symptoms were controlled (Milliren, 1977).

Patients' views of doctors

How do people in general, and women in particular, view the medical services? What are their attitudes to, and how satisfied are they with, the services they receive? These questions can be asked at different levels of abstraction. First, at a general level, views about medicine as an institution, about the medical profession and about the organization and delivery of medical services, can be ascertained. Second, levels of satisfaction with particular kinds of doctors (e.g. gynaecologists, GPs, hospital consultants) can be explored; and third, at a much more specific level, patients' views concerning individual medical practitioners, particular consultations and episodes of treatment, can be collected. Researchers variously have attempted to collect information on these issues, general and specific, which are interrelated, general attitudes to the institutions of medicine influencing specific views on doctors and consultations, and personal experience with individual doctors in turn colouring attitudes to the medical profession and to medical care.

Studies tend to find that at a general level, people have a great regard for Western medicine and medical practitioners. There is an inherent and strong belief in the achievements and accuracy of medicine and considerable deference is accorded to doctors. Even when asked about particular services, such as child health or primary care, the most frequent findings are of general satisfaction from the majority of those asked. It is only when considering relationships with individual doctors, and particular consultations or illness episodes, that criticisms and dissatisfaction emerge.

It has been argued that belief in Western biomedicine has weakened as a result of the publicity concerning medical disasters such as thalidomide, and about the side effects and harmfulness of drugs which previously promised safe solutions to problems (e.g. the contraceptive pill and tranquillizers). Certainly there are indications that drug solutions to problems are becoming less popular, that 'natural' remedies are more sought after, and that 'alternative' medicine has gained ground in recent years. However, it is likely that so far only a minority of, mainly middle-class, people have turned away from traditional medicine and then only in areas where medical knowledge has manifestly failed to provide a solution. Otherwise mainstream thinking continues to adhere as strongly as ever to traditional medicine.

Collecting information about patients' satisfaction with medical services and medical practitioners is beset with methodological problems. Ann Cartwright and her colleagues conducted two interview surveys in England & Wales and found that the majority of people said that they were 'satisfied', or 'very satisfied' with their general practitioners – 91 per cent in the second survey (Cartwright, 1967; Cartwright and Anderson, 1981). Indeed, when people were asked if there were qualities which they thought general practitioners should have, but their doctors had not, three-quarters of the sample could not think of anything to say. It may well be, though, that people who are asked such questions may not have thought about the issues, or may not like to appear critical of doctors. They may have been conditioned to accept medical services in an uncritical spirit and this may well be true of those respondents who habitually feel themselves powerless on encountering the dominance of the medical profession.

Unlike findings in large surveys, small-scale studies which explore patients' views in greater depth, in concrete situations, tend to find a great deal of dissatisfaction with medical services and with individual doctors, and find also that patients are able to say a great deal concerning their reasons for dissatisfaction (Stimson and Webb, 1975; Cornwell, 1984). Moreover, studies exploring the range of patients' feelings about their doctors, report that such feelings fluctuate according to particular experiences and encounters. Ongoing relationships with doctors are seldom straightforward; a person may like some things about a doctor and dislike others and this complexity of likes and dislikes rarely constitutes an end product which can be called 'satisfaction' or 'dissatisfaction'.

Past researchers did not always systematically distinguish between female and male patients' responses to doctors and although it is likely that responses of both are complex there may well be gender differences. However, their feelings about doctors may well be more important to women, most of whom meet doctors more frequently during their lifetime than do men and who more often consult doctors with emotional problems. It is easier to establish patterns of satisfaction and reasons for fluctuations in feelings where relationships between doctors and patients are long-term and regular, rather than being based on the occasional meeting. Thus, the doctor–patient relationship of women who see their general practitioners frequently, who regularly meet their obstetrician during pregnancy, or who are having on-going treatment by their psychiatrists, are of special interest.

What characteristics do women like and dislike in their doctors? The individual doctor's personality, manners and interpersonal skills matter a great deal; indeed, Ann Cartwright found that when asked about the qualities they appreciate in doctors, the majority of respondents say something concerning the ways in which their doctors look after them (Cartwright, 1967). Women, especially, want a doctor to be accessible (i.e. readily available when wanted), approachable (i.e. can be consulted with all sorts of problems), understanding, sympathetic, considerate and not patronizing (Cartwright and Anderson, 1981; Miles, 1988). Home visits also score when patients consider their doctors' manner of looking after them.

In Britain, where the 'family doctor' has traditionally been a provider of medical care on a long-term basis, many women like an on-going personal relationship with one doctor, who knows the whole family. Studies note that women, more than men, hold it to be important to maintain a warm, personal relationship with their family doctor; they want the doctor to be a friend, whom they can trust, rather than someone who appears a cool, distant, scientific expert with whom the relationship can only be business-like (Cartwright, 1967; Miles, 1988; Roberts, 1985).

In their study of three generations of Scottish women, Blaxter and Patterson (1982) noted some changes between generations; more of the older women than the younger ones valued the friendly 'family doctor', and a long-term relationship with one general practitioner, and disliked impersonal service. However, for both older and younger women, the doctor's manner of looking after patients was of the utmost importance.

According to Blaxter and Patterson (1982, pp. 164–165):

For younger mothers, the distinguishing feature of good or bad medical practice was willingness to make house calls. A 'good' doctor was one who came promptly. 'I 'phone back of nine she's here by ten. I never have to wait', and a 'bad' doctor was one who was 'not that ready to come in', or 'takes too long to arrive'.

And (pp. 166–167):

The amount of time the doctor had to spare for a consultation was a salient feature of service for both generations. Grandmothers, particularly, defined a 'good' doctor as one who could offer his time, and a 'bad' doctor as one who 'has the prescription written out before you've even spoken!'.

Patients are not necessarily able to distinguish between the effects of the doctor's personality and manners on the quality of service, and the effects of the structure on that service. Impersonal care, meeting a large number of 'faceless' doctors, the 'conveyor belt' system of seeing patients, are frequent complaints in antenatal care, but these feelings of depersonalization derive as much from the service structure as from the way doctors behave. Thus, women may see many different doctors during pregnancy (Oakley, 1981), and even if each of them is warm and friendly (and the possibility is that some are not) the women experience lack of continuity and the lack of a personal interest in them, factors which may effect their view of doctors.

It is interesting to note that when talking about satisfactory and unsatisfactory aspects of medical care, people very rarely mention clinical aspects of doctors' work: very seldom are references made to the doctor's knowledge of medicine, diagnostic and treatment skills, or medical competence (Cartwright and Anderson, 1981; Roberts, 1985). Even those who talk readily about their doctors' interpersonal skills or thoroughness, do not mention medical capability (Jefferys and Sachs, 1983). It may be that people take doctors' professional knowledge and skills for granted, assuming that these are inherent in medical qualifications, and that lay people do not feel themselves able to judge clinical competence. On the rare occasions when criticism of clinical aspects of the doctor's work is expressed, for example in comments about unhelpful medicines or inadequate examinations, the doctor's errors are attributed to lack of attention, overwork or to dismissing the complaint as unimportant – not to lack of medical knowledge (Stimson and Webb, 1975). In specific cases a doctor may be deemed not to have specialist knowledge: for example, in one study, women, treated by their general practitioners for depression and anxiety and eventually referred to psychiatrists, took the view that general practitioners lacked skills to treat their particular complaints (Miles, 1988).

In view of the dissatisfaction and criticism expressed by many people when talking about the ways in which doctors look after them, how can it be explained that large surveys repeatedly report respondents as saying that they are 'satisfied' with the service they receive? As mentioned before, attitudes are complex and not necessarily consistent. The prestige of medical knowledge and the medical profession is high even if individual doctors are criticized; moreover, the service provided tends to be accepted as not only 'satisfactory', but the only possible service, (where awareness of alternatives is lacking). Commenting on the high proportion of people in her survey who expressed satisfaction with general practitioners, Ann Cartwright took this to be a sign not so much of a positive feeling that everything was well, but of a passive, rather apathetic acceptance of the *status quo* (Cartwright, 1967). There is also an inclination in many people to keep to the 'known' and well-tried, rather than to opt for an 'unknown' service. As Santayana remarked, habit is stronger than reason.

A good illustration of such conformist attitudes is given in a study of women's responses to antenatal care in Scotland, carried out by Maureen Porter and Sally Macintyre. Women's views concerning two types of antenatal care were explored: for women with pregnancies deemed to be 'unproblematic' and where the medical expectation was that the birth would be 'uncomplicated', there were fewer routine visits; more care was provided by GPs and midwives and less by obstetricians, and women were not undressed and palpated at each visit. By contrast, women who were deemed to have 'problematic' pregnancies were seen as often as obstetricians and GPs thought necessary (Porter and Macintyre, 1984). Overall satisfaction and the particular likes and dislikes of women were elicited in interviews. Not surprisingly, in view of previous research, it was found that the majority of women expressed overall satisfaction with the care they received. It was more surprising to find that as between GP surgeries and hospital an almost identical proportion of women, 84 per cent and 83 per cent, respectively, expressed satisfaction (Table 6.1).

In the view of the researchers (Porter and Macintyre, 1984, p. 1198), the

data suggests that pregnant women – and the same may be true of other health service users – are fairly uncritical and assume that whatever care they are receiving has been well thought out and is probably the best there is. These women tended to accept and be satisfied with whatever care arrangements they experienced and to prefer them to alternative possibilities. They were conservative in the sense of saying that 'what is, must be best'.

Table 6.1 Overall satisfaction and usual place of care: percentage of women

Overall satisfaction	Usual place of care	
	GP (n = 164)	Hospital (n = 42)
Dissatisfied	1	5
Mixed feelings	15	12
Satisfied	84	83

Source: Porter and Macintyre, 1984.

Similar 'conservative' sentiments were noted by Ann Cartwright in relation to childbirth arrangements (Cartwright, 1979). However, Porter and Macintyre argued that 'whether it is because of conservatism, deference or politeness that women express preferences for familiar systems of care' such sentiments should not be 'construed as indicating "real" levels of satisfaction' (Porter and Macintyre, 1984, p. 1200). Indeed, women in Aberdeen, where the study was conducted, when interviewed about their likes and dislikes concerning antenatal care, mentioned a number of things about hospital provision that they wished were different; they wanted shorter waiting times, more continuity of care, and a less impersonal atmosphere.

Do women prefer female doctors?

Adults enter upon a consultation with a set of expectations which will include some preconception of what sort of person the doctor is likely to be. Such anticipations are learned in childhood, reinforced in maturity and greatly influenced by gender. Sex-role stereotypes, i.e. generalized ideas of what it is to be a woman or a man, influence expectations of male and female doctors. Thus, because the components of the female stereotype include a nurturing aptitude, expectations of a female doctor may include kindness, caring and understanding. Conversely, widely held stereotypes would lead people to expect a cool, competent-looking, non-demonstrative, authoritarian male doctor. Such, and other expectations, would influence patterns of help-seeking, choice of doctor and satisfaction with care.

There is little information on patients' expectations of female and male doctors. In a study conducted in a United States clinic, private patients' perceptions of doctors of both sexes were investigated (Shapiro *et al.*, 1983). Male and female doctors were perceived as behaving differently towards patients. Women patients expected female doctors to have both interpersonal and technical skills and male doctors to be equipped only with technical skills.

It may be expected that in countries like the United States or UK, where the traditional doctor figure is male, general attitudes would show a preference for male doctors; indeed, that there may be prejudice against female doctors. However, the reality is not so straightforward. In a study, based on the American Medical Association survey of physicians, Langwell (1982) analyzed patterns of patients' demands for the services of male and female doctors (indicators of 'demand' being the number of days patients had to wait for routine appointments, fees charged, etc.). They noted a higher demand for female doctors, who had more patients, and a longer waiting list for appointments.

For women, the gender of gynaecologists and obstetricians is of particular importance. Consultations with these specialists necessarily include undressing and internal pelvic examination and thus are particularly sensitive. Consultations are also likely to include references to potentially embarrassing and very personal topics. Of course, women for generations have been treated by male gynaecologists and obstetricians and possibly have come to perceive them as genderless healers; but it has to be borne in mind that the majority of women had no choice in the past (and hardly more now) because no female specialist in female problems was available. Thus, even if women accepted male obstetricians as 'best' they did so in the context of a situation which provided little or no choice.

Physicians, also, examine women, indeed general practitioners can be called upon to deliver babies and handle sensitive parts of the body. In an interesting study, Susan Ackerman-Ross and Nancy Sochat noted that women preferred female physicians, the preference being most marked when the consultation concerned some kind of sexual dysfunction or when the examination necessitated intimate exposure; they were less marked in their preference when their complaint was, for example, a sore throat (Ackerman-Ross and Sochat, 1980). Male patients who participated in this study also expressed a strong preference for same-sex (i.e. male) physicians when consulting for sexual or otherwise potentially embarrassing conditions.

In British general practice, there have been indications of women favouring female physicians for gynaecological problems, cervical smears tests and, especially, for contraceptive advice, other than the pill (Gray, 1982; Preston-Whyte et al., 1983). Possibly, women expect that a female doctor will have a better appreciation of the feelings of a patient at the receiving end of a gynaecological examination. Indeed, there is accumulating evidence that many women, even those who profess to be satisfied with male doctors, would choose a female obstetrician, were one available. Studies conducted on Well-Woman Centres and Clinics find that one of the main motivations of clients is the assurance of finding female specialists providing the service (King, 1987).

There studies suggest that far from seeing doctors as asexual beings, patients are keenly aware of their doctor's gender, or at least become so when consulting for 'sensitive' matters.

Finding a female doctor may be even more important to the women of certain ethnic minority groups. Considerable literature is now available showing the difficulties experienced by women of a variety of ethnic minority groups in Britain and the United States in their encounters with the medical services of these countries. Cultural and religious beliefs prevent many women of Asian origin from submitting to an examination by a male doctor without a relative accompanying them, while others would not submit to a physical examination by a male doctor at all. Hilary Homans found that 69 per cent of the Asian women she interviewed wanted a female doctor to examine them during their pregnancy. The option to have a female obstetrician can be vital to some women (Homans and Satow, 1981; Homans, 1985).

An interesting aspect of patient preferences is that women who had previously dealt with female physicians and obstetricians seem to be more likely to express preferences for them than are women who in the past dealt only with male doctors (Engleman, 1974). Here again, women have been socialized into accepting male superiority in science and medicine and so to expecting men to be better doctors. Only on experiencing medical care provided by female doctors does patients' confidence in them grow. For example, Haar et al. (1975) found that while 34 per cent of women in their study preferred female gynaecologists, 59 per cent of those who were patients of female physicians, did so. Some writers argue that prior experience of female doctors makes these practitioners more 'credible' in the eyes of patients, thus increasing preferences for them (Weisman and Tetelbaum, 1985).

Preferences for female gynaecologists and obstetricians by women who otherwise are not particularly concerned whether the doctor is male or female, indicate that preferences are situational, that is, specific to the consultation and the particular problem. Further evidence is provided by the preference sometimes expressed by women for male doctors when psychiatric and emotional problems have to be discussed. This preference may not be very widespread, but it has some significance since it might be expected that when women wish to talk about emotional problems, their relationships with their husband, children or parents, causes of depression or anxieties, their preferred choice would be a female doctor. It can be argued that women doctors share the female experience and thus are better able to empathize; and that when problems are connected to the experience of being a house-wife, or a mother, or to biological events such as miscarriage, childbirth or menopause, a woman doctor would be better able to understand and care for female patients.

However, some women appear to have had bad experiences with female physicians and psychiatrists and complain of their lack of sympathy, of their being 'too hard' and of their inability to understand. According to Miles (1988, p. 130):

The psychiatrist was a woman and I couldn't talk to her. She was not married and she didn't understand about husbands and children . . . she didn't have the experience. Her life-style was completely different from mine. For example, she asked me why I thought I had to cook every day, why this was important to me. She didn't understand, she asked silly questions like this.

And

My doctor is a lady doctor and she is very unsympathetic. I can feel it when I try to tell her anything . . . she thinks I am a nuisance. Once she said it was time I sorted myself out. I wish I could change her for a man; they are more sympathetic. Women can get very hard when they have a career.

According to Roberts (1985, p. 17):

I'd always sooner have a man doctor, and now you're going to ask me why. Well, in most cases, I think they're more sympathetic, and I find it easier to talk to a man than to a woman . . . most women are tougher with women.

Trying to account for male doctors being preferred by many middle-aged women in her sample, Helen Roberts (Roberts, 1985, p. 18) argued that

it is culturally more acceptable to appear 'weak' in front of a man, and perhaps, when visiting a woman doctor, there is always the feeling that she also has children to look after, a husband, a home, problems of her own. What is more, that recognition is coupled with the fact that she is there in the surgery doing a job – emphasizing, perhaps, the fact that some women can cope.

It is also possible that stereotypical notions of female doctors as likely to be sympathetic and understanding, raise expectations too high, so that a professional approach disappoints. By contrast, a moderate amount of sympathy from male doctors, from whom a clinical approach is expected, is the more appreciated for being unlooked for.

It may also be the case, however, that women doctors are, in some instances, less sympathetic than their male counterparts, especially towards women who complain of emotional problems and who appear to need not medicine but support. Women in medicine have to be tougher than men in order to succeed (Young, 1981) and, having fought many battles themselves, may lack patience with women whom they regard as unwilling to fight.

Expressed preferences for female doctors are not necessarily translated into actively choosing them. In Britain, people seldom choose their doctors according to gender, or indeed, according to other characteristics such as qualifications; rather, general practitioners tend to be selected by personal recommendation on moving to a new area, or are 'inherited' from childhood, while in some cases no effective choice is available (e.g. rural areas may be covered by one practice only). In the case of specialists, patients are likely to be referred to the nearest general hospital and given little, if any, information on the available specialists, perhaps on the assumption that such information may not always be meaningful to them. However that may be, women are routinely referred to gynaecologists or psychiatrists without choice or explanation. In many areas of the United States and Canada more active selection is possible than in Britain. Kelly (1980), investigating patterns of choosing doctors in San Diego, noted a tendency among patients, both female and male, for choosing doctors of their own sex. Of course, men are better placed to exercise such a choice than are women, female doctors being much fewer in number.

Women's attitudes to health visitors, midwives and nurses

Of the many professionals who provide health care it is the health visitors, the midwives and the nurses, besides the doctors, whom most women encounter and form opinions on, since most women have recourse at one time or another to the maternity and childcare services. As with attitudes to doctors, the approach, manner and personality of these other professionals and the way in which they look after those in their care greatly influence women's views on them. A brusque or a friendly approach by, say, midwife or nurse can be enough to change a previously held attitude (Blaxter and Patterson, 1982; Clark, 1984).

However, some of the views expressed by women about health visitors and midwives indicate that relationships with these professionals is on a different plane than relationships with doctors. Women who express negative attitudes towards health visitors and midwives often accuse them of advising, indeed of interfering, without personal experience of pregnancy and parturition. Some health visitors and mid-wives are, of course, themselves mothers, but many are not and their advice, for example, on what to do during childbirth or how to look after a baby, if based on professional training and not on personal experience, may be resented (Blaxter and Patterson, 1982, p. 168).:

> My last health visitor had no children of her own, so I don't know how she would know. They maybe get trained, but I don't think it's the same as having a baby and doing it.

And Cornwell (1984, p. 194):

> I never went to the classes, so I never found out if the women who give the classes have ever had children . . . If the woman's sitting there and she's never had kids and turns round and says to me, 'Now, if you do this it'll be easier' then I would actually turn round and say, 'well, how the hell do you know if you've never had a baby? How do you know it's going to make it easier?' They can only go by what they're told. . . .

At the core of such sentiments is the view that what health visitors and midwives are able to provide is not professional, expert opinion, but essentially common-sense, lay advice, and in that, the knowledge of women with personal experience is valued over book learning. Indeed, health visitors, antenatal classes and baby clinics are most popular with first-time mothers: those with experience feel much less need for these services with their second and subsequent babies.

Similar views are expressed about social workers and nurses, and, to a much lesser extent, about doctors, respect for medical knowledge ensuring more deferential attitudes. However, it is interesting that doctors are most likely to encounter the attitude that experience is more important than book learning within the maternity services (Cornwell, 1984), possibly because these services deal with a process seen as natural, rather than as sickness.

In Britain, another distinctive feature of women's relationships with health professionals, other than doctors, is the widespread confusion as to which profession they belong and the precise nature of their expertise. Especially, women who encounter several kinds of profes-sional helpers are often vague as to the differences between them, such has been the finding of several studies (Blaxter and Patterson, 1982; Martin, 1989). Women respondents in East London, interviewed by Jocelyn Cornwell, typically displayed this confusion (Cornwell, 1984, p. 182):

> The term 'social work' was used indiscriminately to mean proba-tion officers, almoners, the medical and nursing staff of mother

and baby and child health clinics, health visitors, and district nurses, as well as social workers employed by local social services. The medical and nursing staff mentioned were also frequently referred to as 'welfare workers'.

Health visitors, social workers and community nurses, all appear to offer support and a chance to talk over family matters, so that the dividing line between them becomes blurred and all are consigned by the recipients of their services to the category of generalized helpers: only the doctors stand out.

The social distance between women patients on the one hand and health visitors, nurses and midwives on the other hand is less marked than that between patients and doctors. Women who have positive attitudes towards the 'other' professional helpers often emphasize that they are more approachable than doctors, and that it is easier to relax and talk to them (Miles, 1988). The setting of meetings with them is less formidable: doctors are encountered in consulting rooms and hospitals which can appear strange and intimidating places, whereas health visitors and community nurses provide assistance in the familiar setting of the home.

There is now an increasing number of male nurses and health visitors but little research evidence on how women feel about them. Numbers of male midwives are also increasing and of the mothers interviewed by Ann Oakley, the majority, 70 per cent said that they had no preference for either female or male midwife while 27 per cent preferred a female. However, unless the increase in male midwives is matched by an increase in female obstetricians, the chance of having a female professional assisting a woman at childbirth becomes even slighter.

Conflict and power imbalance in interaction

Differences in expectations, goals, and values, of women patients and of the many providers of health care, are likely to lead to interaction characterised by conflict. Indeed, Eliot Freidson (Freidson, 1975a, p. 286) argued that conflict is inherent in the relationship of patients and health professionals:

> It is my thesis that the separate worlds of experience and reference of the layman and the professional worker are always in potential conflict with each other. This seems to be inherent in the very situation of professional practice ... while both professional worker and client are theoretically in accord with the end of their relationship – solving the client's problems – the means by which

this solution is to be accomplished and the definitions of the problem itself are sources of potential difference.

Professionals and patients may well have different objectives: for example, patients, at the start of a consultation with a doctor, may want a particular prescription, a referral to a specialist, an opportunity to talk over problems, reassurance, a sickness certificate, or a diagnosis. The doctor may or may not think the patient's goal to be appropriate.

Professional workers view the subject of the consultation from a perspective learned during professional training; they are detached from the patients' problems, to which they apply their professional expertise. By contrast, patients experience their individual problems subjectively and view them from a lay perspective. Thus there is a built-in conflict at the heart of the consultation process, which is not to say that it invariably manifests itself. When conflict does arise, the professionals are the likely winners, the two participants in the interaction not being possessed of equal power; professionals, especially the doctors, are, so to speak, in the driving seat. Doctors have the medical knowledge and skills and the access to medicines and services, which puts them in a position of strength. Patients, by contrast, are in an inferior position; they need the doctor's advice and may be weakened as a result of illness. The balance of power is on the side of the doctor, and this is further emphasized by the symbolic significance of the consultation taking place on the doctor's own territory (surgery), where the doctor controls the length of time that the consultation may take, the examination performed, and the outcome of the consultation, e.g. prescription, referral, etc. The appointment system and the period of waiting serve to emphasize that the doctor's time is more important than that of the patient. Asymmetry in relationships is even more marked when the patients come from relatively powerless sections of society, e.g. the working class or ethnic minority groups. Women patients generally have to accept being regarded by doctors as inherently weak and complaining, their time and activities less important than those of male patients. This is emphasized by male doctors' expectations that women will be submissive, and the willingness of many female patients to be so. Thus, the usual consultation between doctor and female patient is not an interaction between equals, nor is it seen to be by either of them.

The power position of patients *vis-à-vis* health professionals, other than the doctors, is somewhat different. These professional workers have less authority than doctors and patients perceive them as being more on their own level. Nevertheless, these professionals are not without power and women often see them as a potential threat. For example, mothers of young children often mention that health visitors and community nurses have the right to 'report' families. According to Blaxter and Patterson (Blaxter and Patterson, 1982, p. 169):

> It was very notable that a high proportion of our respondents volunteered the view that one of the functions of the health visitor – perhaps the major one – was to police child neglect or child abuse . . . one mother described health visitors as 'interfering in some ways, but they find out a lot of child battering that way!'. Others described the health visitor's function as . . . 'to see they weren't being starved. They wouldn't let you starve them!' . . . 'to see your house is clean and tidy for a baby to be in – if you had any family problems I suppose they would report it!'

Similarly, a fear experienced by women who receive treatment for depression and other psychiatric complaints is that health visitors or social workers may deem them to be 'non-coping' mothers and remove their children (Miles, 1988).

Professional–patient conflict and the management of childbirth

Conflicts and power imbalance have been major concerns of researchers and women's movement writers exploring relationships between gynaecologists, obstetricians and their patients. Health professionals working in the field of gynaecology and obstetrics deal with all the functions and malfunctions of the female reproduction system and thus their crucial importance in the lives of women can hardly be overstated (Ruzek, 1978; Scully, 1980).

Conflicts surrounding the management of childbirth have been the focus of many studies and the concern of women's consumer groups. Health professionals and pregnant women view childbirth differently, their views being based on their 'separate worlds of experience and reference', as Freidson pointed out. Doctor and patient would agree on the ultimate goal, the production of a healthy baby! However, other goals of childbirth (for example, the mother's sense of joy and achievement, the control of pain and the process of bonding between mother and baby) may not be equally important to, or even shared by, doctor and mother. Two kinds of expertise, lay and professional, conflict here – the professional, based on general rules and categories, learned during training, and the lay, built up from personal experience and that of the social group.

Perhaps the most serious conflict is over control: who decides important issues such as where the childbirth is to take place, how much technology will be used and whether and when medical intervention is to be resorted to? Hilary Graham and Ann Oakley (1986), on the basis of studies in York and London, reported that women had very few choices about these issues and were unable to exercise control over the kind of childbirth they were to have. Mother's lack of control has been confirmed by numerous British, U.S. and Canadian studies (Oakley, 1981; Romalis, 1985). When there is a clash, the doctor's superior power ensures that the patient gives in. Open and visible conflicts are rare, not because women are satisfied with medical control but because they feel themselves too powerless to oppose it. In this, women have much right on their side. The setting of childbirth has shifted from home to hospital, and in the hospital labour ward the patient is in no position to exercise control. Fear of punitive measures ('they will just leave me and no-one will come') and fear of the sedative ('just a jab to make me quiet and I'll not know anything') are usually adequate to ensure the patient's acquiescence.

The wishes of pregnant mothers concerning the management of childbirth are by no means consistent. On the one hand, many women would like to have more control themselves, medical intervention and the use of technology only if essential, and a less clinical, more personal atmosphere. On the other hand, women have been repeatedly told by obstetricians and other health professionals that technological childbirth is safer childbirth, and have come to believe that the 'experts' know best.

Several researchers have found that women want more say in how childbirth is managed; many are not in favour of intervention, in the form of forceps delivery, epidurals and induction. Even when accepting · the desirability of some medical procedures, for example, foetal heart monitoring, women point to their undesirable effects on their experiences (e.g. restricting movement during labour) (Oakley, 1981; Graham and Oakley, 1986). The BBC consumer programme *That's Life!* in 1982 presented the replies to their questionnaire about the experience of childbirth (Karpf, 1988). The overwhelming response of women showed their wish for more choice in the style of labour and their view that childbirth is not a mechanical process to be managed by doctors.

However, television broadcasts in Britain during the 1980s gave contradictory messages: consumer programmes sought to influence mothers against technology during childbirth, but other programmes glamorized hospital birth. Anne Karpf explained that there were many programmes on childbirth during the 1980s because (Karpf, 1988, p. 76)

> to TV producers in general, birth was an attractive subject, highly telegenic. It was dramatic, emotional, and generally had a happy outcome. It wasn't illness, but could still mobilise the glamour

of doctors and hospitals. It was also a visible, infinitely filmable event, happening in hours or days, rather than a slow invisible process, and since all of us have been born and most women still give birth, it had wide audience appeal.

It would be misleading to suggest that all women wish to oppose obstetricians' control. Describing the negotiations between obstetricians and pregnant women in Canada, Shelly Romalis argued that (Romalis, 1985, p. 186)

In this technological era women have come to believe that having a baby is a complicated and dangerous affair, that all kinds of physical and emotional problems can arise, often at the eleventh hour, making prediction impossible. It is therefore necessary to have a highly trained expert on hand to locate and manage these problems when they occur.

Many women's acceptance that birth should be in a hospital and that the use of technology is desirable, has been influenced by obstetricians who convey this message with all their power and authority.

Even in matters where there is general consensus among women as to desirable practices, the chances of their being successfully achieved, in the face of opposition or indifference by professionals, is slim. Most women would agree that freedom to move around during the long hours of labour is desirable and that medication rendering one unconscious for delivery is undesirable (Sullivan and Beeman, 1982). Yet, in practice, movement is often controlled and medication often given and there is hardly anything a women in a labour ward can do to protest. Freidson's point that patients may be physically weakened when facing the doctor, would certainly apply to a woman in labour who wants kindness and not conflict.

However, to argue that the balance of power is tilted towards doctors is not to argue that patients are completely powerless. Consumer groups are able to achieve changes that are hardly within the scope of individuals; patients have some control through financial arrangements and in rather extreme cases doctors are vulnerable to the displeasure of patients. Few general practitioners would care to be in a position where every patient who comes to the surgery says 'I would see any doctor except Doctor X.' Patients have some control in that they are not obliged to go to any particular doctor (although changing from one to another can be far from easy), nor are they obliged to follow doctor's recommendations. Indeed, this is why obstetricians are in a particularly powerful position amongst doctors: pregnant women cannot escape their sphere of influence, or escape procedures ordered by them. It is somewhat different in consultations between general practitioners and patients between whom interaction is not only a conflict but also a negotiation, where doctor and patient struggle, from their different perspectives, to reach common ground (Stimson and Webb, 1975; Bloor and Horobin, 1975).

The problem of information

When people express dissatisfaction over their encounters with health professionals, one of the most common complaints concerns the lack of access to information (Stimson and Webb, 1975; Cartwright and Anderson, 1981; Jeffreys and Sachs, 1983). There is widespread dissatisfaction with the amount of information received from professionals, mainly doctors, concerning all aspects of diagnosis, prognosis and treatment.

Although dissatisfaction comes from women and men, working class and middle class, the extent of the information obtained from the doctor varies according to social class and to gender. It has been argued that rapport between doctor and patient is easier to achieve if they are of similar background and status, or the social distance between them is small. A male doctor may communicate better with a male, professional patient than with a female or working class patient. Information-giving may be more effective where there is greater rapport: doctors are likely to be more willing to provide explanations if they feel confident that the patient understands and if they have a high regard for the patient. Certainly, research in Britain suggests that it is the working class patients who receive the least explanation (Cartwright and O'Brien, 1976). In a study where consultations between general practitioners and patients were tape recorded, Tuckett and his colleagues found that social factors influenced the information patients received. For example, doctors were less likely to give clear explanations to Afro-Caribbean patients than to others (Tuckett *et al.*, 1985).

Women fare rather worse than men as several studies, analysing tape-recorded consultations, show. For example, Wallen *et al.* (1979) found that doctors gave shorter answers and less technical explanations in reply to questions posed by female patients. Tuckett *et al.* noted that women were twice as likely as men to have their ideas 'evaded' by doctors and Fisher and Groce (1985) showed that female patients categorized as 'bad women' were less likely than others to get full replies to their questions.

Lack of information is closely linked to powerlessness. Decisions can only be made on the basis of information and if a woman is not properly informed about the diagnosis or treatment of her condition, her chances of making meaningful decisions are diminished. It is, in any case, a humiliating, even frightening, experience to learn that other people know more about one's body, health and future than oneself, and are able to refuse the disclosure of vital information. It is humbling for an adult to be placed in the position of a child and told not to ask questions. The following quotes came from women in maternity care (Oakley, 1981, pp. 283–284):

> If they give you your notes to take somewhere they give them to you in a big sealed brown envelope stapled up, and if you want to read them you have to get them down from the rack in the cubicle and you get caught . . . The staff nurse came in and said 'Oh, you mustn't read these' and she got very cross. She said 'You're much better off if you don't know anything'.
>
> . . . They don't like you reading your form . . . They leave your notes lying about in that cubicle thing. The nurses tell you off. One doctor did find me, he said 'Do you find it interesting?' I said, 'Well, it's my form, I'm not going to look at someone else's'.

Another area of complaint among women is that health professionals withhold information regarding the side effects and after-effects of treatment. Professionals may prefer not to warn about possible adverse effects because they do not want to frighten patients, but to experience worrying symptoms without prior warning is unpleasant. In one study, hysterectomy patients said (Webb, 1986, p. 101):

> I would have liked a bit more information. Half the problem is worrying about it and not knowing.
>
> I think they should warn about complications. It would give you some warning so that you know it can happen or it's nothing to worry about.
>
> If somebody had told me that I might see a lot of blood I would not have been so frightened . . . I think they should tell you that you might have a complication or infection or lose a few drops of blood – then you wouldn't worry so much.

Again, women who have tranquillizers prescribed for them by their doctors are known to complain that possible side effects are not explained, leaving them to find out when things go wrong (Miles, 1988). Patients seldom think that doctors are unaware of side effects and possible complications; the assumption is that professionals choose not to warn about such possibilities.

Explanations are also felt to be too few when medical procedures are carried out in hospitals. Women often complain that in maternity wards the staff do not tell them why certain procedures such as putting up a drip, ultrasound monitoring, or repeated urine testing, are carried out (Kirke, 1980).

Referrals to a specialist can be made without the patient being told of the reason and full information about the prognosis is by no means always made available to patients. The usual assumption of the women concerned is that health professionals are too busy to spend time on explanations or that they think patients would not understand; some even think that professionals deliberately conceal information. Researchers suggest that health professionals, especially doctors, give little information not because they want to conceal, but because they lack the skills to explain (Cartwright, 1967; Jefferys and Sachs, 1983). Certainly, it seems from research that even when doctors are in favour of being frank and informative, patients feel that what they are told is inadequate (Kirke, 1980). Lack of information also results in patients' acceptance of what is done to them and fits in with the medical view of interaction in which the patient is a passive recipient of the service.

However the situation comes about, lack of information reduces women's ability to understand and to make choices, for example, whether to have the treatment or not. 'The right to choose' is an important and often repeated demand of the women's movement because in the economic sphere and elsewhere women have fewer choices than have the men. Further reduction of choices, through lack of information about their health and what is being done to them in the name of health, adds to women's lack of power.

If patients want more information, why do they not ask? It is the consistent finding of research that patients, both women and men, are reluctant to ask questions and, if they do not understand an explanation, reluctant to say so. The reason for reluctance is that patients feel actively discouraged by health professionals and lack the confidence to assert themselves. It can be humiliating, especially for women whose self-confidence is low, to have to indicate their lack of understanding, and to feel that the professionals regard them as ignorant (Graham and Oakley, 1986, p. 64):

> The nurse says, 'Now do you want to ask the doctor anything?' and more invariably than not you say, 'No', because you just don't feel you can. The way they ask you, 'Right, do you want to ask the doctor anything?', you think, 'No'. All you want to do is get up and get out.

Doctors may, of course, express information in highly technical language which patients are unable to understand. To patients this can seem deliberate exclusion and in some cases it is. For example, Graham and Oakley (1986) noted that doctors used technical words to pregnant women when they wanted somewhat unwilling patients to agree to particular procedures. However, the employment of such terminology can also be the result of professional training where clinical knowledge

Table 6.2 Ability to speak English in minority communities (1976)
(percentages)

Standard of English	Pakistani		Indian		East African Asian	
	Men	Women	Men	Women	Men	Women
Fluently	28	8	43	22	56	33
Fairly well	29	11	28	15	21	34
Slightly	35	36	19	36	14	22
Not at all	8	41	7	24	5	19
Not stated	1	2	4	3	3	1

Source: Mares *et al.*, 1985.

is expressed in highly technical language. Professionals may be unable to translate esoteric knowledge into language which is accessible to lay people. The result is to mystify patients and exclude them from informed decision-making. There are, in addition, other sorts of difficulty. Women whose cultural background and first language is different from that of the health professionals experience special problems both in asking for information and in understanding it. Technical and colloquial explanations, tone of voice, conventions of politeness and ways of structuring information may all have different meanings in different cultures. (Thus, for example, Homans found that pregnant Asian women would prefer to say, 'I feel weak' instead of 'I think I am pregnant' to their doctor; (Homans and Satow, 1982).)

Table 6.2 shows the respective percentages of women and men who speak English among some minority groups, living in Britain, whose first language is not English. It is the women of these groups who have the greater language difficulties, the proportions of them who cannot speak English being considerably higher than the corresponding figures for men. Learning the English language is far from easy as the following quote from a teacher of English as a second language, illustrates (Mares *et al.*, 1985):

> There's a lot of blame attached to people who can't speak English, and of course it's very, very frustrating for health workers. They can't do their job properly and the reason is the patient's inability to speak English. But sometimes I feel that if they themselves ever tried to learn another language, as adults I mean, or if they'd ever taught English and seen what hard work it is to learn a foreign language, they might be a little more tolerant. After all, let's face it, the person who really suffers is the patient who can't speak English.

Not all women are treated in the same way and not all feel themselves equally powerless to demand information. English-speaking, White, well-educated, middle-class patients are the most likely to obtain information and be given it in straightforward language, while working-class and non-White women may meet condescension. (For example, student nurses relating instructions they received in a maternity hospital, said that if patients seemed educated and 'able to understand', they were told to use terms such as 'internal examination', 'vaginal examination', or 'induction', but where patients were expected not to understand, such terms were replaced with 'examination down below', 'feel inside you', or 'give the baby a push'.)

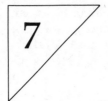

The medical control of women

A recurring theme of the preceding chapters has been that the interpretation of moods, feelings and bodily sensations as potential or actual illness, and encounters with medical services, loom large in the daily lives of women. It has been argued that medicine affects women more than it does men because a greater part of the female experience comes into the medical orbit. This is not a situation which is 'inherent' or 'natural', thus requiring no explanation; on the contrary, it is important to consider why and with what consequences women's lives come so much within the purview of health professionals and medical structures.

The influence of medicine in women's lives has been increasing during the second half of this century, a fact not entirely to be seen in the context of medical expansion in general.

The medicalization thesis

From the early 1970s several writers drew attention to a trend for the expansion of the sphere of medicine in Western societies. This trend, referred to as 'medicalization' was described by Irving Zola (Zola, 1975, p. 170) who argued that

medicine is becoming a major institution of social control, nudging aside, if not incorporating, the more traditional institutions of religion and law ... this is not occurring through the political power physicians hold or can influence, but is largely an insidious and often undramatic phenomenon accomplished by 'medicalizing' much of daily living, by making medicine and the labels 'healthy' and 'ill' relevant to an ever increasing part of human existence.

Subsequently, others have argued that an increasing emphasis on the prevention of disease, and on 'healthy' habits and life-styles, shifts medicine into the lives of healthy people. Balanced diet, the amount of exercise taken, leisure activities, type of housing and heating, alcohol consumption, cigarette smoking, standards of cleanliness, body weight, all come under medical scrutiny in the name of disease prevention. As early as 1971, Zola contended that under certain conditions virtually any human activity and habit can become medical concerns as specially trained health professionals become deemed to have expert knowledge on how people should live and conduct themselves (Zola, 1971). As this process takes hold, the emphasis on prevention and health consciousness grows. In Britain, government and health professionals more and more stress not only that prevention is better than cure, but that prevention is 'everybody's business' (DHSS, 1976). Thus, health promotion and health education have come to be important activities as individuals are given to understand that they have a social responsibility to lead a healthy life and to combat disease. The arbiters on what constitutes a healthy life-style, and the expert advisers on how to prevent disease, are the health professionals, whose opinions are sought on an increasingly large number of issues.

Expansion of the orbit of medicine is continuing in other ways as well. As medical technology becomes ever more sophisticated, and pharmaceutical companies bring new products on to the market, so does the inclination to make use of these improvements expand also. Abnormalities can be detected, and potential diseases treated before they occur. So, acceptance in affluent Western societies that not only life but the quality of life are the legitimate concerns of medicine means that the wishes of individuals to be slimmer, or taller, or more attractive and to stay youthful, fall into the sphere of medicine in the belief that new technology and new drugs can help towards the desired end. Nor is this trend confined to medicine: in the wake of the doctors an ever-growing number of other health professionals are now on hand, stressing their own expertise and ready to give guidance on a whole range of 'good practices' from bringing up baby to keeping fit in old age. As these 'other' professionals receive a more prolonged and higher level of education and training, and their organizations grow in stature, so does the requirement to find a market for their newly-acquired knowledge and skills among one or other client group, grow also.

Another area of medicalization which has attracted the attention of social commentators is that of 'disapproved behaviour'. Freidson argued that many, if not all, kinds of disapproved behaviour have been shifted into the realm of medicine and re-interpreted as sickness rather than the previously accepted label of 'crime', 'badness' or 'sin'. Quoting examples such as heavy alcohol consumption, redefined as alcoholism, and shoplifting as a symptom of mental disturbance, Freidson (Freidson, 1975a, p. 249) argued that:

The medical mode of response to deviance is thus being applied to more and more behaviour in our society, much of which has been responded to in quite different ways in the past. In our day, what has been called crime, lunacy, degeneracy, sin and even poverty in the past is now being called illness, and social policy has been moving toward adopting a perspective appropriate to the imputation of illness.

Critics of the trend increasingly to medicalize areas of daily life have pointed to the role played by health professionals in social control. The medical profession's role as an agent of control was described by Talcott Parsons (1951) in his essay on the sick role and subsequently was critically analysed by several writers (Szasz, 1961; Freidson, 1975a; Zola, 1975; Conrad, 1979). The thrust of their argument is that the medical profession functions to ensure conformity to social norms. More than that, the profession is influential in establishing norms of behaviour and uses medical means to eliminate or minimize behaviour which deviates from such norms.

Thomas Szasz argued that doctors were, in the past, involved with conditions relating to the structure and function of the human body, but that later they focused on disabilities and suffering of all kinds (Szasz, 1961, pp. 44–45):

Then, with increasing zeal, physicians and especially psychiatrists began to call 'illness' anything and everything in which they could detect any sign of malfunctioning, based on no matter what norm. Hence, agoraphobia is illness because one should not be afraid of open spaces. Homosexuality is an illness because heterosexuality is the social norm. Divorce is illness because it signals failure of marriage.

When the label 'illness' is applied to some type of behaviour, what follows is 'treatment' as prescribed by health professionals; when doctors define standards of health, health-promoting activities, and behaviour harmful to health, they establish norms and it becomes their function to control behaviour in a way that ensures conformity. According to Friedson (Friedson, 1975a, p. 250):

The consequence of the movement is the strengthening of a professionalized control institution that, in the name of the individual's good and of technical expertise, can remove from laymen the right to evaluate their own behaviour and the behaviour of their fellows – a fundamental right that is evidenced in a hard-won fight to interpret the scriptures oneself, without regard to dogmatic authority, in religion and the right to be judged by one's peers, in law.

Not all doctors wish to expand the boundaries of medicine and many are opposed to particular areas of expansion. Indeed, Conrad (1979, 1981) has pointed out that medicalization and controlling behaviour in the name of health, can occur without either the active participation or the wish of medical professionals. Certain groups, for example Alcoholics Anonymous, can adopt medical ideology; courts of justice sometimes insist on a medical opinion; state welfare authorities often demand medical co-operation. All effectively extend the control function of medicine without the doctors consciously seeking to exercise this function, although they no doubt enjoy the enhanced prestige which attends the expansion of medical boundaries.

There are checks on the growth of medicalization. Strong (1979) pointed out that financial constraints can be severe in times of tight state control of spending on medical (and other) services. Thus, increasing medicalization of, say, old age, is deterred by lack of willingness to increase the burden on tax payers (Macintyre, 1977 b).

Writers on medicalization and control have given little attention to the differential effects thereof on various sections of the population. On women, the impact of the growth of medical influence has been very considerable: in particular, three aspects of the increasing medical control of women's lives will be discussed in the following pages, namely the interpretation of women's difficulties and unhappiness as psychiatric problems, the medicalization of female biological processes, and the intervention of health professionals in the spheres of childcare and family care.

Women and psychiatric control

Epidemiological studies have shown a preponderance of females among those diagnosed as suffering from psychiatric problems. As discussed in Chapter 1, information on treated patients comes from hospital admission statistics, data gathered from general practices, and from community samples. Available information shows especially high rates for neuroses and affective disorders in women. Smaller gender differences are recorded for psychotic illness (such as schizophrenia) and for organic conditions such as senile dementia. The gender distribution is reversed in personality disorders (e.g. psychopathy) and in conditions involving misuse of drugs and alcohol, where males dominate. However, these latter categories form only a small percentage of all psychiatric illnesses.

The greatest gender difference is in conditions which are usually dealt with by general practitioners without reference to psychiatrists and which, if referred to psychiatrists, are treated on an out-patient basis. Also, there is some evidence of considerable gender differences in problems experienced, but not diagnosed and treated; this is the conclusion of surveys carried out by professionals assessing the volume of symptoms which would receive treatment if brought to doctors. The Cambridge *Health and Life-style Survey* (Cox *et al.*, 1987) investigated psycho-social symptoms in a sample by asking questions about anxiety, sleeping patterns, concentration, fatigue, and related items, and found that such symptoms were significantly greater among women. It was noted that a third of the females in the sample attained a threshold score at and beyond which, according to the measure employed, there is a possibility of psychiatric disorder being present.

How does it come about that so many more women than men experience problems which are defined as psychiatric and for which they receive treatment from doctors? Is this an indication of the growing trend of medicalization? Is the implication to be drawn one of an increased medical control of women?

There are two perspectives, two ways of looking at the question of why women are prone to becoming psychiatric patients. One is that women experience stresses and hardships to a greater extent than do men and are, literally, 'driven mad' by oppressive social structures. The other is that women are more likely than men to be labelled 'neurotic' or 'mad' by professionals and lay people, due to the widely-held female stereotype of the neurotic, complaining woman and because of women's relative lack of power to reject the application to them of adverse labels. These two perspectives have much in common with the 'social causation' and 'artefact' explanations of higher rates of female morbidity (see Chapter 1) but they are not synonymous with them.

Both perspectives have their exponents and many interesting and lively debates have appeared in the pages of books and journals during the last twenty years.

That women experience more stresses in their lives and resultantly have more mental illness, was argued by Walter Gove and his colleagues in a number of papers (Gove, 1972, 1978; Gove and Tudor, 1973). In their work, they focused on women's psychiatric illness and marital status and adduced epidemiological evidence to show that married women have more mental illness than do married men. Mental illness is slightly higher in single men than in single women, but the numbers are much smaller here, as most of the adult population is married. Stresses in the lives of married women who spend their days, mainly in the company of children, in the confines of the home, have been much discussed. Several studies demonstrate the plight of women who are engaged on full-time domestic work, many of whom suffer from frustration, boredom coupled with fatigue, loneliness and low self-esteem, lack of independence and lack of power (Oakley, 1974; Sharpe, 1984; Land, 1981). Those who also have jobs outside the home, although they may gain in companionship, self-esteem and a measure of independence, find additional sources of stress as they try to function as 'good' employees as well as 'good' mothers and wives, working even longer hours and suffering further frustration, guilt and physical exhaustion (see Chapter 1). Women's experiences are well documented, and the link between stress, hardship and frustration on the one hand, and mental illness on the other, has been promulgated by many investigators (Chesler, 1972; Oakley, 1981; Busfield, 1983; Rosenberg, 1984). Especially can this link be argued for anxiety disorders and neurotic conditions, where research evidence indicates the presence of social aetiology. George Brown and his colleagues identified a number of social factors which contribute to depression in women (Brown and Harris, 1978). Brown divided these social factors into 'provoking agents' which triggered the onset of depression and 'vulnerability factors' which made women more susceptible to this disorder. Among provoking agents, certain kinds of adverse events in the lives of women (such as bereavement, serious illness, accident, marriage breakdown, etc.) were found to be important, while ongoing difficulties (e.g. poor housing, the threat of eviction for non-payment of rent, drug-taking in the family) also served to provoke depression. Vulnerability factors were the lack of close, confiding relationships with husband, relatives or friends, the loss of mother early in life, lack of paid employment outside the home coupled with the presence of young children (especially under six years of age) in the home. Elsewhere, it was found that in close communities social factors, such as the oppressive nature of closeness and lack of opportunity to escape from it, increase women's vulnerability to anxiety disorders (Brown *et al.*, 1977).

Thus, there is much support for the influence of social factors in the causation of anxiety disorders and depression and it can be argued that the reason for women having higher rates of these conditions lies in their unsatisfactory lives. More thorough analysis is needed, however, before any assertion that mental illness generally is linked with the broader structural features of society. (For a review, see Busfield, 1988.)

The second perspective on women and mental illness contains the argument that women are more likely than men to be labelled 'mad' or 'neurotic'. This line of thinking draws on the work of critics of psychiatry (the so-called 'anti-psychiatry' school), and on the labelling theorists (Szasz, 1961, 1971; Scheff, 1966; Laing, 1967; Wood, 1983). The most systematic application of the labelling perspective to mental illness can be found in the work of Thomas Scheff, who noted that mental disturbance may arise from many diverse causes (some biolo-gical, others genetic, psychological or social): what is common in psychiatric patients is that they, in some way or other, break social rules, and become labelled as mentally ill. Scheff argued that the act of being so labelled is the most important thing that happens to the individuals concerned. He also pointed out that mental disturbance is a socially constructed category, which can only be understood in a situational context (e.g. loud laughter may be taken as a sign of merri-ment or madness, depending on the situation). Scheff and other critics of psychiatry also maintained that psychiatry is very powerful (this, indeed, has been noted about medicine as a whole) and that psychi-atrists have more power over their patients than other medical practition-ers have over theirs. (This argument needs to be treated with caution. In England recently, children have been forcibly taken into care and families placed under severe strain, following allegations by doctors of child abuse.) Psychiatrists' power includes the giving of compulsory treatment, and the taking away of the liberty of individuals; the fact that these powers are seldom exercised in late twentieth century West-ern democracies and then only in extreme cases, still leaves in place the potential threat. (A look at the 'treatment' given, quite recently, by psychiatrists to dissidents in oppressive regimes, makes clear the potentially dangerous power of psychiatry and the possibility of abuse.)

Critics further allege that psychiatric practice does not always work in the interest of the patients, any more than medicine in general does. For example, Ivan Illich (1977) made the point that doctors generate needs while making sure that only they can supply the remedies. From a Marxist perspective, Navarro (1976) argued that doctors fit their medical services to the needs of a capitalist society and not necessarily to the needs of individual patients. Psychiatry then can serve the interests of the state, and of the profession, as well as, or in preference to, that of the patient. Critics also say that at least some psychiatric labels should be abandoned, because they serve no useful purpose. According to Wood (Wood, 1983, p. 48):

For many thousands of years the human race has done without this concept of neurosis and must and will learn to do so again.

That we have a word for it does not explain what it is, if it exists or what, if it truly exists, is the best thing to do about it. The concept of 'neurosis' has not helped the plight of 'neurotics'.

The arguments of the critics of psychiatry have been considered specifically with regard to female patients, and also further developed, by feminist writers. In her influential book, *Women and Madness*, Phyllis Chesler (1972) viewed psychiatry not only as an oppressive, but as a male oppressive enterprise, dominated by men who adhere to traditional stereotypes of female inferiority and weakness. Chesler argued that psychiatrists devalue female behaviour and see women as psychiatrically impaired and unbalanced. Other writers pointed out that male healers in general, and not just psychiatrists in particular, tend to define women's emotional problems and sufferings as sickness (Smith and David, 1975; Ehrenreich and English, 1979; Barrett and Roberts, 1978). Psychiatrists work with formally established diagnostic categories; but when they diagnose a patient, cultural expectations as to what is healthy and what is sick behaviour influence their judgements. To Scheff's observation that 'odd' or 'rule-breaking' is meaningful only in a situational context, should be added that what constitutes 'appropriate' behaviour is different for men and for women. Thus, Joan Busfield (Busfield, 1988, pp. 533–534) argues that:

Defining excess fear as pathological is not neutral as to gender in a culture where expressions of fearfulness are more acceptable amongst women than men, since women are more likely to manifest all degrees of fearfulness. Simply by acting in ways considered more appropriate to their gender women are closer to and more in danger of being phobic than men. The same is true of depression and anxiety, since the expression of these emotions is considered more appropriate in women than men.

It can thus be argued that under current psychiatric practice, women are more likely than men to be labelled as psychiatrically ill because female role prescriptions in society place them closer to the kind of behaviour that psychiatrists see as neurotic, phobic or depressed. Besides, if psychiatrists, like some other doctors, find women demanding, complaining or in other ways unsatisfactory patients (see Chapter 6), negative views may be translated into negative labels, such as 'neurotic woman'.

Phyllis Chesler (1972) suggested that women who do not conform to the female gender stereotype are also vulnerable to psychiatric labelling. Housewives and mothers who complain of frustration and are unhappy at home; women who show hostile feelings to husband or children; those who appear more aggressive, less submissive, or less patient and kind, than the stereotype leads people to expect, may also be called 'unnatural' and even 'pathological' by professionals. The general stance is that 'normal women don't behave like this, you must be crazy'.

It is not only psychiatrists who put such labels on women (although they are best placed to do so); other professionals and lay groups may act similarly, and for similar reasons. Stereotype expectations are strongly held and medical views are pervasive, influencing lay and professional thinking. In a study of patients of a mental health centre in the United States, Horwitz (1977) found that women there were more likely than men to be labelled by friends and relatives as having psychiatric problems, a factor which may channel women towards psychiatric services.

Implicit in the writings of feminist authors on this subject is the assumption that a psychiatric label is a negative one, with some damaging consequences. Leeson and Gray argued that a diagnosis such as 'neurotic', when applied to women, is a hostile label: 'From the way the term is used, you might think it is not so much a diagnosis as a moral failing – and we suspect it is often used like that' (Leeson and Gray, 1978, p. 159). The consequences of receiving a psychiatric diagnosis could be beneficial in that counselling and treatment appear to be of value with certain kinds of affective disorder. However, much of the literature suggests that labels like 'neurotic', 'anxious' or 'depressed' may have more negative than positive consequences. Certainly, it is possible to argue that women have higher rates of psychiatric illness because of differential labelling.

The two perspectives, i.e. that women's negative experiences make them more vulnerable to mental distress and that women are more likely than men to be labelled as psychiatrically ill, are not mutually exclusive. On the contrary, it is likely that they are correlative, that depression and anxiety in women are essentially social phenomena, rooted in the social structure which shapes their lives, and that the ways in which women become defined as psychiatric patients are also social in nature and are linked to the power of psychiatry and the powerlessness of women.

The consequences of psychiatric labelling and treatment

The woman who finds herself beset by a sea of troubles, who is unhappy and 'failing to cope' is likely to turn, eventually, to the medical enterprise where she may well be given a psychiatric label and be offered a medical solution for her problems. Viewing this process at the doctor–patient interaction level, it seems that the two participants actively collude in medicalizing the woman's problems. How does this come about and what are the consequences?

It is easy to understand why a woman turns to a doctor with her emotional, social or family difficulties: there may not be anyone else to turn to and the doctor may be the only person who can offer immediate relief. Struggling with an alcoholic husband, caring for a senile parent or a handicapped child, feeling frustrated and unhappy because a career was given up in favour of childcare, are not medical problems. But they can become so, once they cause, as they inevitably do, sleeplessness, worry, fatigue and mental exhaustion. The doctor can give immediate, albeit temporary, relief, by prescribing pills which induce sleep or which lift depression. By consulting doctors, women medicalize their unhappiness and frustration.

Taking problems to doctors has an additional benefit. Certain kinds of unhappiness and frustration cause tremendous guilt feelings; women feel guilty about failed marriages, troubles with children, for not doing even more for their aged or sick relatives, or for not being super-mothers and wives (Miles, 1988). A medical explanation reduces the guilt: if failure, real or imagined, or even an inability to be happy can be attributed to illness, the individual feels the personal blame lightened. Unfortunately, the benefits brought by imputing problems to illness, are dearly bought.

Before looking at the price women pay, the question arises as to why doctors are willing to accord psychiatric labels to complaints which appear to have little or no recognizable medical basis. Individual doctors, whether general practitioners or psychiatrists, have much pressure on them to provide 'treatment' for unhappiness. Friedson (1975a) argued that doctors are trained to be positively helpful to patients, i.e. that they have an 'activity orientation', and do not like to send patients away empty-handed. Doctors feel better if they can make a diagnosis and provide a treatment for complaints, otherwise they may feel a sense of inadequacy for the task. As one psychiatrist put it, speaking of patients who come for treatment, 'we feel we should bend over backwards to provide it. It makes us feel better if we do, worse if we don't.' (Wood, 1983, p. 30).

Increased emphasis on prevention during the 1980s also put pressure on doctors to provide treatment and support for unhappy, frustrated, struggling patients, in order to forestall the possibility of mental disorder. Richman and Bury (1985) in a paper entitled 'More and more is less and less: the myth of massive psychiatric need', argued that psychiatrists increasingly accept for treatment patients with a whole range of 'socio-behavioural' problems. These patients are not exclusively women but it is the women who, for reasons discussed before, receive more medical attention and psychiatric labelling.

Pressure on doctors to assign patients to a diagnostic category arises because treatment can only follow if a diagnosis is made. As there is no diagnosis called 'unhappiness' or 'socio-behavioural problem' doctors use what Scheff called the 'dustbin' category of medical diagnosis: depression, anxiety or neurosis.

What, then, are the consequences for women of receiving one or another psychiatric label for their problems? One consequence is that many of the women so labelled are given a prescription for some psychotropic drug (e.g. tranquillizers, sleeping pills or antidepressants), indeed general practitioners have little else to offer to patients with psycho-social problems. During the 1970s, much concern was expressed about the so-called 'over-prescribing' (a rather curious term, as if there exists a level of prescribing which is neither 'over' nor 'under' but exactly right) of psychotropic drugs and this focused especially on women receiving such prescriptions, as it was noted that, in several Western countries, more than twice as many women than men received these drugs (Choiton *et al.*, 1976; Hemminki, 1974). There is some evidence that fewer prescriptions for psychotropic drugs were issued during the 1980s as doctors became more aware of the side effects and addictive propensities of these drugs (Hemminki *et al.*, 1981; Koumjian, 1981). However, even if the overall level is falling, the gender differences remain.

The harmful effects of tranquillizers and antidepressants are well known and women who take these preparations tend to be disparaging about them (Miles, 1988). The pattern seems to be of the usefulness of these drugs when first prescribed, followed by diminishing confidence in their benefits when used long term. Side effects can also be a problem. A major difficulty which follows reliance on drugs for lengthy periods (addiction) is trying to come off them. Some typical comments of drug-taking women are worth quoting (Miles, 1988, p. 132):

> I couldn't think straight, it's as though my mind was blocked off. I forgot everything I was so tired. When I stopped taking them I could think again, I was alert and remembered things.

> Valium isn't the answer but by the time you find out you can't give it up. Doctors don't know what withdrawal means, they don't believe me when I try to explain. Even the loss of one tablet can be a disaster.

Thus, psychotropic drugs are seldom an unmitigated benefit for women who use them. From a broader perspective, giving a psychiatric label to distress and seeking to alleviate it with drugs, is open to criticism. The effect of the process is that the underlying causes of

women's unhappiness are ignored, especially where they are rooted
in the social structure, and women are maintained in frustrating and
oppressive situations. The controlling function of psychiatry becomes
evident: giving women psychiatric labels and pharmaceutical preparations ensures that they are able to continue in domestic roles or
as care-providers. Cooperstock and Lennard (1979) in their study of
Canadian Valium users noted that such drug-taking functioned to
maintain women 'in a role which they found difficult or intolerable
without the drug', and that, typically, was the domestic role.

In their study of female patients, Michele Barrett and Helen Roberts
(1978) argued that general practitioners and psychiatrists aimed to
'adjust' women to their painfully endured domestic roles (Barrett and
Roberts, 1978, p. 42).

> In consultation after consultation the G.P. smooths away the
> surface anxiety and adjusts the women to the limitations of a life
> located totally in the home ... the institution of medicine legiti-
> mates and endorses the *status quo* in relation to the position of
> women, and in so doing it fulfils an ideological function as an
> agency of disguised social control.

The researchers found that general practitioners diagnosed as 'psychosomatic' complaints, women's boredom, frustration or listlessness.
Others have noted that the most frequently-given reasons for taking
Valium are tension, to keep calm, anxiety, or to relax (Caplan *et al.*,
1985). But neither doctors, nor women patients, examine the roots of
women's difficulties, or question the structure in which they flourish.

Viewing women's unhappiness in a psychiatric perspective and
labelling it psychosomatic, results in minimizing the problems and
discrediting the women who complain. Thus, current psychiatric practice sends a dual message, firstly, by locating the problem in the
personality, ability or adjustment of the female patient and regarding it
as individual inadequacy, and, secondly, by assuring the patient that
she is ill and cannot help being maladjusted, unable to cope, or inadequate. Women receive the dual message in the form of psychiatric
diagnosis and explanation. Beside the old and well-worn labels of
depression and neurosis, there are others which are increasingly used
and accepted, and which illustrate the problematic nature of medicalizing women's unhappiness. One such is 'pre-menstrual tension'.

The prevalent view of pre-menstrual tension is that it is caused by
hormone imbalance, particularly imbalance of the hormone progesterone, which is said to cause changes in fluid balance leading to changes
in the brain and, in turn, to severe mood changes (Birke, 1986). The
assumption is that the mood fluctuations and the distress that women
complain of are determined by hormones and advocates of this theory

have found that treatment with progesterone sometimes helps sufferers. Lynda Birke points out that no consideration is given to the
possibility that life-style or diet may affect hormone production; the
determinant is assumed to be the hormone itself, and women are made
to seem helpless in face of their own biology.

Post-natal depression

Unhappiness, anxiety, despair, frustration and helplessness approach-
ing panic, are variously experienced by many women during the weeks
and months following childbirth. Health professionals call these sensations 'baby-blues' or 'post-natal (or post-partum) depression', and tend
to attribute them to hormone-changes associated with birth and breast-
feeding. It is important therefore to explore the consequences of viewing mothers' negative feelings in a medical framework. The first question to ask is whether such feelings are commonly experienced and a
number of studies have attempted to provide an answer. Ann Oakley
(1981) divided post-natal problems into three categories: having 'blues'
while still in hospital, experiencing anxiety state on going home, and
other depression at home. According to her study based on talking
with women, 84 per cent of mothers had hospital 'blues', 71 per cent
anxiety at home and 24 per cent other depression. Other studies,
concerned only with identifiable psychiatric conditions, recorded lower
percentages; thus, Kumar and Robson (1984) noted 14 per cent 'de-
pressive neurosis' in women in the first three months after childbirth,
while Paykel *et al.* (1980) found that 20 per cent of mothers had 'mild
clinical depression' at six weeks after birth.

Unhappiness, however, expressed, is certainly very real for many
mothers who might reasonably have expected the arrival of a new baby
to be a joyous event. Especially after a first baby, but also after subsequent ones, the mother must adjust to a new domestic situation, to
playing a new role and to forging new relationships to replace those
which might be lost. She may have to contemplate the loss, or at least
the interruption, of her career and with it a loss of freedom and
economic independence. Suddenly the home seems too small, her
husband is on edge and the baby cries all night. All these things crowd
in upon a woman who may be physically weakened by childbirth
and worried by her inexperience. Respondents in Oakley's study said
(Oakley, 1981, pp. 143–145):

> I think I was terribly affected by the whole thing. I was really
> surprised at that – the whole thing about adjusting. I was just
> miserable, tearful, crying at everything, at the slightest thing . . . I

just felt so miserable and at night she wouldn't go back to sleep and I just was beside myself. I just wanted to die.

I kept thinking that I'd never be able to cope with him and do anything else at all... that's something I never want to go through again, that couple of weeks, it was a terrible feeling. I don't know whether it was reaction because I'd had a rough time and I was still probably tired.

I just felt so drained myself, I got feelings of panic, I felt so uptight in my stomach and I looked around me and I thought gosh, there's no-one here who can cope with her.

Negative feelings, despair and exhaustion may well be connected with bad childbirth experiences. Oakley and others suggest that women whose labour is heavily technological and those who undergo a prolonged childbirth of which they are not in control, are the more likely to be depressed and unhappy afterwards. Moreover, lack of support and practical help on a daily basis, after going home from hospital, can also produce negative reactions, as feelings of being alone to cope with all that the new baby means and of immense responsibility for another life, become overwhelming. Oakley (1981) suggested that when the woman's mother is present to provide daily help and support, and to relieve the isolation, any so called 'depression' can be nipped in the bud. Paula Nicolson (1986) found in her study that the changes in relationships brought about by a new baby can mean that the mother drifts away from her husband and loses his support instead of gaining more. One of her respondents said (Nicolson, 1986, p. 144):

I am not completely happy... I cry a lot, almost every day. My husband is confused and probably fed up, and a barrier is coming up between us. I can see it, but I can't stop it.

Others have observed that strained marital relationships and lack of support are linked with post-natal unhappiness and negative feelings (e.g. Paykel *et al.*, 1980). In contemporary society, many women are isolated from their female kin group; in the case of first babies, many prior friends are lost because relationships were with childless women on a basis of freedom to come and go. Husbands (or male partners) are then the only available sources of support. However, cultural expectations dictate that spouses share in each other's lives so that the mother of a new baby expects the father to be interested in the newcomer. When the reality is otherwise, it is all the more painful for being unexpected. When marital conflicts emerge, or worsen, the isolation of the woman is intensified. Hopkins (1980) suggested that husbands can be 'stress factors' for women after childbirth.

Other social factors also can affect women's mental state at this time: difficulties with housing, a variety of stresses such as family conflict, were noted in this context (Paykel *et al.*, 1980; Kumar and Robson, 1984).

There are, then, a wide variety of reasons for a woman to be unhappy, anxious, and frustrated, at a time when social expectations are that she should be glad. When she is not, yet another emotion awaits her, a sense of guilt: 'I must be an unnatural mother' is a typical distressful reaction.

Given that hormone changes are a normal bodily response to pregnancy and that the adverse sensations experienced by new mothers are rooted in social causes, then to what extent can a medical label and medical treatment be said to be appropriate? Within a relatively short time 'post-natal depression' has become an established category of disorder (Oakley, 1986), and health professionals talk about it without questioning its validity. Yet critics argue otherwise. 'Post-natal depression is not a "scientific" term but an ideological one. It mystifies the real social and medical factors that lead to mothers' unhappiness.' (Oakley, 1981.)

In the present social structure, many women are understandably unhappy when they struggle, in isolation, with a demanding baby. This feeling is widespread, as Ann Oakley found, and indeed, health professionals assure women that 'blues' and post-natal depression are to be expected: advice literature for mothers constantly relays the message that it is normal to be depressed (Oakley, 1986). Yet, the use of medical terminology, such as 'post-natal depression' or 'post-partum depression', implies that this 'normal' condition is, after all, a medical one, and that the appropriate experts to manage or treat it are the health professionals. The message inherent in medical terminology is that women should not rely on their own experiences or on those of other women, but should be advised by health visitors, midwives or doctors.

Some women may suffer from an identifiable psychiatric condition, although even here such a condition may well be rooted in the current social structure. But many others struggle with problems in their lives which may be amenable to social solutions, and are unhappy because they have every reason to be. Medicalizing their problems by the attachment of psychiatric names and guiding them towards health professionals obscures the nature of their problems. Questions concerning problems embedded in the social structure are not asked and there is little chance of solutions. As with 'depression' and 'anxiety' in women in general, the task, as seen by professionals, is not to find radical solutions, but to 'adjust' the mothers of young babies to their unhappy situations.

Medicine and female reproductive processes

Pregnancy and childbirth, of all the female reproductive processes, became most completely medicalized in the second half of the twentieth century. Several writers have documented the history of the process whereby childbirth was transferred from the private domain of the home to the public domain of the hospital, from its management by lay females (i.e. experienced women) to control by (mostly male) professionals, and from its being a 'natural' biological event to a highly technological, medical, one (Donnison, 1977; Arney 1982; Oakley, 1984a).

A woman, finding herself pregnant, finds also that a regime of antenatal care is laid down for her, that she is expected to report regularly during pregnancy to a clinic or surgery and undergo medical checkups and tests, and that quite early in the pregnancy arrangements are made for the birth to take place in a particular hospital or nursing home, where she will duly go to have her baby delivered under professional supervision and with whatever medical monitoring and intervention is thought appropriate. Elsewhere in this book the interpretation of pregnancy as health or illness (Chapter 2), and women's views about childbirth and professional control (Chapter 6) have been discussed.

So pregnancy and childbirth are not in the process of being medicalized: they are already. From the day a woman's pregnancy is confirmed until after delivery, what she eats and drinks, how much she works, exercises, and rests, all become the concern of health professionals. In the name of health, not only her own but with even greater emphasis that of the foetus, the activities of the pregnant woman are controlled and so is her labour and the delivery of her baby. It is now illegal in most Western countries for an unqualified person to deliver a baby, and in the vast majority of cases delivery takes place in a hospital or clinic.

Other parts of the reproductive process have not been so completely medicalized, however, but an increase in medical control is currently taking place. One example is the medicalization of the menopause, which is all the more interesting because it brings into the medical orbit a large area of the life of middle-aged women, just as the medicalization of pregnancy has done in respect of younger women.

The term menopause refers to the final cessation of the menses; however, in both medical and lay language it is used more broadly, usually to include some time before and after this event. This timespan can be prolonged, beginning with the months during which the menstrual cycle becomes increasingly irregular, until the year after the last menstruation during which there is the possibility of another menstrual period. The timing for most women is for all this to occur between the ages 45–55. Although the process is a natural part of the life cycle, there is a great deal of medical concern with possible malfunctioning, how to deal with it, and how to prevent its occurrence.

Susan Bell (1987) argued that medicalization of the menopause began seriously in the late 1930s and early 1940s, basing her argument on an analysis of papers in medical journals by members of the 'medical elite' of North America. In 1941 a synthetic oestrogen became available and this marked the beginning of oestrogen replacement therapy. Once available, this therapy offered the possibility of treating all menopausal women, not only those with bad symptoms, and in this way all became potential patients. Indeed, in current medical literature, especially in the United States and Canada, the menopause is regarded as an 'oestrogen deficiency disease' which can be treated by replacement therapy. So defined and treated, the menopause changes from being a normal biological process to being a health problem, even a disease.

Endocrinology research has identified lower oestrogen levels during the menopause; the only set of symptoms clearly linked to this decrease in oestrogen are hot flushes and sweats, troublesome symptoms for some (although not all) women and for which therapy replacing the lost oestrogen certainly appears to be the answer. According to Susan Bell, it seemed logical to medical specialists to do something about lower oestrogen levels (Bell, 1987, p. 538):

> In a lecture to the New York Academy of Medicine, Robert T. Frank, Clinical Professor of Gynecology at the College of Physicians and Surgeons (Columbia), compared the treatment of menopause to the treatment of two deficiency diseases. In his view, 'the estrogenic relief of the menopause' was 'a major triumph, second only to the treatment of hypothyroidism by thyroid medication and of diabetes by insulin!' In other words, menopause, like hypothyroidism and diabetes, was a deficiency disease and therefore it, too, could be treated with a replacement therapy.

With their condition defined as a treatable physical problem, menopausal women are drawn into the medical orbit; they are encouraged by doctors to seek medical advice with their symptoms and discouraged from relying on lay experience. The menopause, as a problem which produces symptoms, becomes defined as 'bad' in the sense that disease is bad, instead of being seen as a normal phase of the life cycle (Frey, 1981).

Hot flushes and sweats at night constitute not only discomfort by themselves, they may also lead to further problems, such as sleeplessness, which in turn can be treated, further drawing women into the medical orbit. Moreover, in medical literature, much emphasis is placed on psychological problems experienced by menopausal women. Feelings of insecurity, loss of purpose, depression, and anxiety, have been attributed to the menopause, although the link between biological changes and these symptoms is not clarified. In Britain especially, the 'empty nest' syndrome is much referred to; indeed, an examination of popular family health advice books and medical dictionaries show this to be a constant theme in describing the menopause. The theory is that for middle-aged women who have raised their children and seen them off into the world, the home is like an empty nest with the woman in it experiencing a loss of function, role, usefulness and purpose. Naturally, goes the argument, depression and other psychological problems will follow, to which the medical response can take the form of psychotherapy, psychotropic drugs, or just support and good advice (Bell, 1987).

Patricia Kaufert rightly pointed out that a woman may simultaneously be depressed and menopausal. In a society where menopause is seen in a positive light and defined as symptom-free, neither woman nor healer would attribute her depression to the menopause; only in a society where depression is defined as a possible symptom of the menopause will this attribution occur (Kaufert, 1982). In these latter societies, however, it will occur with a vengeance. A British study of middle-aged women and their doctors, showed that whatever difficulties these women had in their lives, doctors were likely to attribute them to the menopause (Barrett and Roberts, 1978). Women complain that even with symptoms which are least age-connected, doctors tell them 'what do you expect at your age?' or 'it's all to do with the "change" of life' (Roberts, 1985).

Underlying the 'emptying-the-nest' explanation is the assumption that all women live in conventional nuclear families, have children who eventually fly the nest, and that child-rearing is a woman's only interest. This picture may fit some but not all women; women without children and women pursuing careers also go through the menopause and may be depressed for a variety of reasons. Moreover, women who nurse and care for frail, elderly parents, or sick and disabled family members, have no 'empty nest', rather one that is overfull of demanding people.

Medical explanations for the psychological problems and unhappiness of middle-aged women, locate both problem and solution in the individual. Of course, it is likely that some women are depressed or anxious or unhappy quite independently of their menopause; for others, negative feelings about life may well be evoked by the cessation of their menstrual periods. But all this takes place in specific social settings of Western societies where the menopause is negatively evaluated (see discussion in Chapter 4). Medical practitioners, locating problems in the individual, reinforce traditional stereotypes of women as potentially unbalanced by their biological make-up: the menopause, like menstruation, becomes yet another 'proof' that women are vulnerable to hormonal influences.

Not all menopausal women seek medical advice and not all who report their problems to a doctor are given medication or, indeed, treatment of any sort. Kaufert and Gilbert (1986a) carried out a Canadian study of women in the middle years of whom 34 per cent had reported hot flushes to a physician and only 15 per cent had received hormones for this condition. However, no less than 82 per cent of the women studied thought that their physician was or would be helpful to them during the menopause, while 65 per cent of them had actually been given some information on the menopause by their physician. Women who think that health professionals are the appropriate source of information and help concerning the menopause, medicalize the condition, as do those professionals who are willing to act in that capacity (Corbett, 1981).

Several researchers on the use of psychotropic drugs have noted that middle-aged women are relatively high drug users and this has been attributed to problems, social and psychological, surrounding the menopause. However, psychotropic drug use is closely bound up with doctors' views of women and with doctors' prescribing habits, as previously discussed. Kaufert and Gilbert (1986b) on examining psychotropic drug taking in the course of their study in Canada, suggested that it is related to whether a woman's husband or children are causing her problems rather than to their absence from the home. For menopausal women too, as Cooperstock and Lennard (1979) noted, tranquillizers and antidepressants can be the means of adjustment to a life they otherwise find difficult. The possible side effects and addictive qualities of these drugs tend to be disregarded in favour of short-term relief.

Medicalization of the domestic domain

While the most comprehensive and complete medicalization of an arguably non-medical and natural happening has taken place in the field of childbirth, where an identifiable single event could be transferred to the medically controlled public domain of the hospital, medical control is also increasing in the private domain of the home. Medical ideas and models are being adopted in relation to motherhood and marriage, while domestic work is modified to fit in with advice by health professionals. Not only doctors but a growing number of specialist health workers and trained 'helpers' are available with their opinions and advice, backed by the prestige of 'scientific medicine' and designed to promote 'good health'.

Medical influence and childcare

The involvement of doctors in the care of babies and their instruction of women as to the healthy way of bringing up their children, are not new. From the early part of the twentieth century, the prevention of infant mortality and the promotion of child health became the interest of the emerging specialists in paediatrics. The British Paediatric Association was founded in 1928 and doctors specializing in child health came to consider themselves the experts on infant care. They also considered that many mothers, especially working class mothers, were ignorant of baby care and lacking education in looking after young children (Oakley, 1986). However, the proliferation of health professionals, the increase in their statutory duties and the resultant wide surveillance of child health have taken place during the second half of the century. Professionals offer advice and instruction on the 'healthy' and 'right' way of feeding, holding and bathing a baby, on the infant's 'satisfactory' weight gain, growth, and its intellectual and movement development. They know what to do when the baby cries or cannot sleep and have answers ready for whatever other questions may come up. Meantime women's own intuitive knowledge and the accumulated wisdom of the social group become lay, i.e. inexpert, in the eyes of professionals who emphasize that theirs is the only valid and authentic expertise.

The advice of health professionals is offered through leaflets distributed to clinics, in the pages of magazines and newspapers, by television and radio and directly by the professionals to mothers in baby clinics, and doctors' surgeries.

Of course, mothers are not obliged to follow advice and, indeed, some are critical of the professionals. It was mentioned in Chapter 6 that researchers found critical attitudes in women towards health visitors, midwives and social workers who were not themselves mothers. According to Jocelyn Cornwell, many women in Bethnal Green, London, felt that baby clinics are needed only when experienced female advisers (mother or sister) are not available and then mostly for first-time mothers, who lack experience (Cornwell, 1984). The usefulness of school health services was questioned by mothers in Scotland, according to Blaxter and Patterson (1982). Nevertheless, women widely read, watch and absorb medical articles and programmes and frequently act according to popularly disseminated health advice. Indirectly, the thinking of even 'critical' mothers is influenced.

In addition to increasing expert advice on caring for the child's physical health and well-being, medical professionals have also turned their attention to psychological aspects of mothering. During the 1970s, emphasis on 'bonding' between mother and baby first became fashionable. Indeed, in some hospitals obstetric practice changed in order to 'improve bonding', mothers being given the chance to hold their new-born babies (Oakley, 1986). Ironically, health professionals now consider it to be their task to promote bonding not just by discontinuance of the practice of transferring new-born infants to the baby ward, but generally by giving advice to mothers on how to love their babies!

The psychological health and happiness of children is also now a matter for experts, who tell mothers what to do about naughty children, give advice on punishment and reward, unhappiness at school, sibling relationships, and other matters.

An interesting example of the medicalizing of child-rearing is given by Peter Conrad (1981), who traced the establishment and wide acceptance of a new medical diagnostic category, 'hyper-activity'. According to Conrad, although the roots of its discovery go back to the 1930s, it was first described as a disorder treatable with medication by Laufer, in 1957. Symptoms of hyperactivity were given as excess motor activity, inattentiveness, fidgetiness, restlessness, impulsivity, mood-swings, and aggressive-like behaviour. By the 1970s, in the United States, hyperactivity was described as one of the most common child problems, and was treated as such by paediatricians, it being estimated that between 3 and 10 per cent of U.S. children of junior school age could be eligible for treatment. Conrad (Conrad, 1981, p. 117) says that:

> Restless, fidgety children, who do not sit still or pay attention in school and who are often disruptive and difficult to manage at home, have probably always been with us. However, medicalizing hyperactivity is beneficial to important established institutions. Schools now have an effective means of reducing the disruptiveness of such children; families too are less disrupted and parents need not feel guilt as the cause is considered to be organic; pharmaceutical companies who have heavily promoted stimulant medical treatment for hyperactivity, have managed a substantial profit – reportedly $13 million from Ritalin in 1970 alone – from their manufacture, and physicians themselves have another means of 'helping' distressed families with their internal problems.

The main concern of Conrad was to show how disapproved behaviour, in children as well as adults, is becoming the concern of medicine and how social control is slipping into a medical framework and being taken over by doctors. However, the popularity of the diagnostic category of 'hyperactivity' in the United States also illustrates the increasing medicalization of the upbringing of children, and the medical control of motherhood. Naughty, fidgety, inattentive children can be regarded as medical concerns and given treatment. Mothers are told that there is such a thing as hyperactivity, after which they can consider such behaviour in their children as possibly indicating a medical problem. Thus are the thinking and the actions of mothers modified by medicine.

Medical emphasis on the psychological health and well-being of children puts the onus onto mothers who see themselves as primarily responsible for their children. The behaviour of children, defined as 'problem' can be linked to mothers' neuroticism or depression, or to their working away from home, etc. The underlying assumption of health professionals and lay people alike is that the general welfare of the family is the mother's business.

Medicine and domestic work

Although the medicalization of the domestic scene is most apparent in matters of childbirth and childcare, it is not confined thereto. The long-dominant germ theory of disease has its corollary in the belief that cleanliness is an essential prerequisite of disease prevention. The home, where the family spends much of its time, must therefore be clean and to see that it is so falls upon the housewife and mother. What constitutes a 'clean' home is negotiable and in diverse households different standards of cleanliness and tidiness are acceptable, at least to its members. Recent improvements in domestic appliances, aimed at lightening the burden of domestic work succeed rather in raising the level of what is achievable. Health advisers and product advertising combine to exhort women to strive for 'whiter than white' standards, not just in the clothes-wash but in every corner of every room in the house. That lack of cleanliness is tantamount to neglect of children is the message before every mother and the potential disapproval of health visitors and other professionals (to say nothing of friends and relations), is a lurking threat for many housewives.

Food and its preparation have received much attention from dieticians and other specialists. Belief in the merits of good home cooking is not new but it was interesting to have it confirmed in recent British research (Murcott, 1982, 1983), this despite the spread of 'junk' foods and the growth of the takeaway trade. The women seeking to provide adequate and nourishing food for the family is, however, bombarded with medical advice and the advertising of food producers and manufacturers, much of it confusing or contradictory: sugar provides energy but rots teeth; meat and dairy products are natural and healthy but raise cholesterol levels; eat plenty of fresh fruit and vegetables, organically grown for preference; calcium builds bone, or does it? Suddenly bran is promoted because the body needs roughage, at least until this idea is superseded by another, and calories must be counted lest one puts on weight. As if this were not enough, scare stories regularly appear regarding the presence of *Salmonella* or some other organism in this food or that; even water cannot be trusted.

It might be argued that women are not obliged to follow any particular standard of home care and that they can cook much as their mothers did. But social expectations place responsibility for the family's health on the woman of the house and following 'expert' advice enables her to claim that she has done all that she could.

Medicalization of family relationships

Medical ideas, medical practice and advice, permeate the ways in which people today think about relationships within the family. Not only mother–baby bonding, but relationships between wife and husband, and parents and older children are coming to be considered in a medical framework. A range of health professionals offer advice on how to conduct relationships within the family, and many people turn to them for help.

Repeatedly, surveys have found that people consider it appropriate to consult their general practitioner with marital problems and difficulties with their children (Dunnell and Cartwright, 1972; Cartwright and Anderson, 1981). One reason for this could be that other sources of advice and help have weakened or even broken down. For example, in an increasingly secular society, help is less likely to be sought from clergymen and, with greater mobility, older relatives may no longer live nearby. On the other hand, the general practitioners' surgery is easy to locate and usually accessible. However, the vogue for seeking advice and help from doctors and other professionals, while owing something to their availability, reflects also the current thinking of lay people and professionals that there exists a category of adversity variously called 'marital problems' or 'domestic difficulties' for which medical or other professional assistance is appropriate and may legitimately be sought.

'Marital difficulties' and like expressions can be a coded means of describing unsatisfactory sexual relationships; they may also be used to describe the emotional stresses of family life, the division of responsibilities, the personal habits of one partner as they affect the other (anything from snoring to alcoholism), trouble with children or with in-laws, indeed, almost any aspect of life which adversely affects the wife–husband relationship. Increasingly, it is assumed that professionals can provide answers.

Although both partners to a marriage are part of its problems the definition of these problems as potentially medical concerns affects women more than it does men. Women are more likely to think in depth about relationships (Miles, 1988) and to consult professionals. Culturally, women are held responsible for family harmony and their lives are more likely to be centred upon the domestic world of the home, often without another occupation beyond its confines. If professional help is needed, it is the woman who has failed.

An indication of the medicalization of marital problems is that not only counselling but 'therapy' is offered by professionals who define such problems in a medical framework. The *British Journal of Family Therapy* was started in 1979; in the United States, membership of the American Association for Marital and Family Therapy increased from less than 1000 in 1970 to 7500 in 1979; literature on the subject of treatment for the exigencies of married life, by skilled professionals, has proliferated (Morgan, 1985). These professionals are not medically trained and many of them would resent the argument that their work is part of a medicalizing tendency. Their therapy does not involve drugs and hospitals; but the therapeutic approach to marriage implies a view of healthy and of pathological relationships and therapists endeavour to identify marital problems, to locate their sources and to offer solutions. In this broader sense, medicalization means placing the institution of marriage in a framework where the labels of health and pathology are applicable and where trained therapists offer treatment. Moreover, a usual path to marital therapy is through referral by a doctor, and this also places marriage in the orbit of medicine.

Examining some of the literature on marital therapy, Morgan (1985) found therein a 'fairly conventional model of family roles and household structure' (p. 40). He noted that the majority of texts mentioned neither class nor other forms of inequality. Gender differences were most frequently assumed to be biologically based and thus immutable. Morgan also noted 'the adoption of a medical model in marital counselling', and went on to say that 'the very notion of "sexual dysfunction" . . . implies the adoption of a medical model' (p. 47).

For women, the growing medicalization of marital relationships implies more medical control: their culturally assumed responsibility for a happy marriage brings them into the orbit of medical thinking and therapeutic advice on how this responsibility can best be discharged. The professionals' usual aim is to restore the marriage and enable the partners to stay together. Women living in oppressive marriages see therapeutic work as aiming to adjust them to the *status quo*, especially when children are present. Other goals of therapy (e.g. to enable the partners to get on better, to feel happier about the marriage and to achieve better understanding) are also essentially control mechanisms the aim of which is adjustment to bad situations, in the interest of maintaining the structure.

In his review of marital therapy, Morgan (1985) observed that the knowledge on which marital therapy practice is based, derives from a cumulative body of literature on casework. Casework defines and treats individuals without reference to their social ambience and reinforces the view that the problems of marriage are amenable to solution without regard to the worlds of employment, recreation and politics – in short, that marriage is a private concern that exists independently of the wider structure. Inherent in this view is the belief that women's problems are individual and personal and are treatable by recourse to the health professionals.

So it is that medical ideas and practices now pervade wide areas of the female experience, concerning themselves not just with women's general health but also with their natural bodily mechanisms, besides reaching into their jobs and their domestic lives.

Bibliography

Ablon, J. (1981) Stigmatised health conditions. *Social Science and Medicine*, **15B**, 5–9.

Ablon, J. (1986) Reactions of Samoan burn patients and families to severe burns. In Currer, C. and Stacey, M. (eds) *Concepts of Health, Illness and Disease – A Comparative Perspective*. Leamington Spa: Berg.

Ackerman-Ross, F. S. and Sochat, N. (1980) Close encounters of the medical kind: attitudes toward male and female physicians. *Social Science and Medicine*, **14A**(1), 61–64.

Alexander, D. A., Taylor, R. J. and Fordyce, I. D. (1986) Attitudes of general practitioners towards premenstrual symptoms and those who suffer from them. *Journal of the Royal College of General Practitioners*, **36**, 10–12.

Allan, G. (1985) *Family Life*. Oxford: Blackwell.

Anderson, R. and Bury, M. (eds) (1988) *Living with Chronic Illness*. London and Boston: Unwin Hyman.

Arber, S., Gilbert, G. N. and Dale, A. (1985) Paid employment and women's health: a benefit or a source of role strain? *Sociology of Health and Illness*, **7**(3), 375–400.

Armitage, K. J., Schneiderman, L. J. and Bass, R. A. (1979) Response of physicians to medical complaints in men and women. *Journal of the American Medical Association*, **241**, 2186.

Armstrong, D. (1989) *An Introduction to Sociology as Applied to Medicine*. Bristol: Livingstone.

Arney, W. R. (1982) *Power and the Profession of Obstetrics*. Chicago and London: University of Chicago Press.

Baker, R. and Woodrow, S. (1984) The clean, light image of the electronics industry: miracle or mirage? In Chavkin, W. (ed.) *Double Exposure – Women's Health Hazards at the Job and at Home*. New York: Monthly Review Press.

208   *Women, health and medicine*

Balarajan, R., Yuen, P. and Bewley, B. R. (1985) Smoking and the state of health. *British Medical Journal*, **291**, 1682.
Baldwin, S. and Glendinning, C. (1983) Employment, women and their disabled children. In Finch, J. and Groves, A. (eds) *A Labour of Love: Women, Work and Caring*. London: Routledge & Kegan Paul.
Balint, M. (1964) *The Doctor, His Patient and the Illness*. London: Pitman.
Banks, M. H., Beresford, S. A. and Morrell, D. C. (1975) Factors influencing demand for primary medical care in women aged 20–44. *International Journal of Epidemiology*, **4**, 189–95.
Barker, D. J. and Rose, G. (1984) *Epidemiology in Medical Practice*, 3rd edn. Edinburgh: Churchill-Livingstone.
Barrett, M. and Roberts, H. (1978) The social control of women in general practice. In Smart, C. and Smart, B. (eds) *Women, Sexuality and Social Control*. London: Routledge & Kegan Paul.
Bayliss, R., Clarke, C., Oakley, C. M. *et al.* (1986) Incidence, mortality and prevention of infective endocarditis. *Journal of the Royal College of Physicians*, **20**, 15–20.
Beale, N. and Nethercott, S. (1985) Job loss and family morbidity: a study of factory closure. *Journal of the Royal College of General Practitioners*, **35**, 510–514.
Becker, H. S., Greer, B., Hughes, E. L. *et al.* (1961) *Boys in White*. Chicago: University of Chicago Press.
Becker, G. (1981) Coping with stigma: life-long adaptation of deaf people. *Social Science and Medicine*, **15B**, 21–24.
Bell, S. E. (1987) Changing ideas: the medicalization of menopause. *Social Science and Medicine*, **24**(6), 535–542.
Belloc, N. B., Breslow, L. and Hochstim, J. R. (1971) Measurement of physical health in a general population survey. *American Journal of Epidemiology*, **93**, 328–336.
Berkman, L. F. and Syme, S. L. (1979) Social networks, host resistance and mortality: a nine-year follow-up study of Alameda County residents. *American Journal of Epidemiology*, **109**, 186–204.
Bernstein, B. and Kane, R. (1981) Physicians' attitudes toward female patients. *Medical Care*, **19**(6), 600.
Birchmore, D. F. and Walderman, R. L. (1979) The woman alcoholic: a review. In Robinson, D. (ed.) *Alcohol Problems*. London: Macmillan.
Birke, L. (1986) *Women, Feminism and Biology*. Brighton: Wheatsheaf.
Black, J. and Ong, B. N. (1986) Women and health courses: our bodies, our business. In Webb, C. (ed.) *Feminist Practices in Women's Health Care*. Chichester and New York: Wiley.
Blaxter, M. (1976) *The Meaning of Disability – A Sociological Study of Impairment*. London: Heinemann.
Blaxter, M. (1981) *The Health of the Children*. London: Heinemann.
Blaxter, M. (1983) The causes of disease: women talking. *Social Science and Medicine*, **17**, 56.
Blaxter, M. (1985) Self-definition of health status and consultation rates in primary care. *Quarterly Journal of Social Affairs*, **1**, 131.
Blaxter, M. (1987a) Self-reported health. In Cox, B. D. (ed.) *The Health and Life-style Survey*. London: Health-Promotion Research Trust.

Blaxter, M. (1987b) Alcohol consumption. In Cox, B. D. (ed.) *The Health and Life-style Survey*. London: Health-Promotion Research Trust.

Blaxter, M. (1987c) Beliefs about the causes of health and ill-health. In *The Health and Life-style Survey*. London: Health-Promotion Research Trust.

Blaxter, M. (1987d) Attitudes to health. In *The Health and Life-style Survey*. London: Health-Promotion Research Trust.

Blaxter, M. and Patterson, E. (1982) *Mothers and Daughters: A Three Generational Study of Health Attitudes and Behaviour*. London: Heinemann.

Bloom, J. R. (1982) Social support, accommodation to stress and adjustment to breast cancer. *Social Science and Medicine*, **16**, 1329–1338.

Bloor, M. J. and Horobin, G. W. (1975). Conflict and conflict resolution in doctor/patient interactions. In Cox, C. and Mead, A. (eds) *A Sociology of Medical Practice*. London: Collier-Macmillan.

Bott, E. (1957) *Family and Social Network*. London: Tavistock.

Bourne, P. G. and Winkler, N. J. (1978) Commitment and the cultural mandate: women in medicine. *Social Problems*, **25**, 430–440.

Bray, G. (1979) Obesity in America. *International Journal of Obesity*, **3**, 363.

Brenner, M. H. and Mooney, A. (1983) Employment and health in the context of economic change. *Social Science and Medicine*, **17**, 1125–1138.

Briscoe, M. (1987) Why do people go to the doctor? Sex differences in the correlation of G.P. consultation. *Social Science and Medicine*, **25**, 507–513.

British Medical Journal (1980) Women in hospital medicine. *BMJ* **281**, 6242.

Brockman, J., D'Arcy, C. and Edmonds, L. (1979) Facts or artifacts? Changing public attitudes toward the mentally ill. *Social Science and Medicine*, **13A**, 673–682.

Brown, A. (1986) Coping with Agoraphobia. PhD thesis, University of Southampton.

Brown, G. W. and Harris, T. (1978) *The Social Origins of Depression*. London: Tavistock.

Brown, G. W., Harris, T. O., Maclean, U. *et al.* (1977) Psychiatric disorder in London and North Uist. *Social Science and Medicine*, **11**, 367–377.

Brown, G. W. *et al.* (1986) Social support, self-esteem and depression. *Psycological Medicine*, **10**, 813–831.

Brunel ARMS Research Unit (1983) *Discovering the Diagnosis of Multiple Sclerosis*. General Report No. 3. Brunel University.

Burnell, I. and Wadsworth, M. (1981) *Children in One Parent Families*. University of Bristol, Child Research Unit.

Burnfield, A. (1985) *Multiple Sclerosis: A Personal Exploration*. London: Souvenir Press.

Burstein, A. (1981) Curiouser and Curiouser. *The Pharos*, Summer 1981, p. 14.

Bury, M. (1988) Meanings at risk: the experience of arthritis. In Anderson, R. and Bury, M. (eds) *Living with Chronic Illness*. London and Boston: Unwin Hyman.

Busfield, J. (1983) Gender, mental illness and psychiatry. In Evans, M. and Ungerson, C. (eds) *Sexual Divisions: Patterns and Processes*. London: Tavistock.

Busfield, J. (1986) *Managing Madness: Changing Ideas and Practice*. London: Unwin Hyman.

Busfield, J. (1988) Mental illness as social product or social construct: a contradiction in feminists' arguments? *Sociology of Health and Illness*, **10**(4), 521–542.

Byrne, P. S. and Long, B. E. (1976) *Doctors Talking to Patients: A Study of the Verbal Behaviour of General Practitioners Consulting in their Surgeries.* London: HMSO.

Calnan, M. (1984) Patterns in preventive behaviour: a study of women in middle ages. *Social Science and Medicine*, **20**, 263.

Calnan, M. (1987) *Health and Illness – The Lay Perspective.* London and New York: Tavistock.

Calnan, M. and Johnson, B. (1985) Health, health risks and inequalities: an exploratory study of women's perceptions. *Sociology of Health and Illness*, **7**(1), 76–93.

Caplan, R. D., Cobb, S., French, J. R. *et al.* (1975) *Job Demands and Worker Health.* Washington: US Department of Health, Education and Welfare.

Caplan, R., Andrew, F., Conway, C. T. *et al.* (1985) The social effects of diazepam use: a longitudinal field study. *Social Science and Medicine*, **21**(8), 887.

Cartwright, A. (1967) *Patients and their Doctors – A Study of General Practice.* London: Routledge & Kegan Paul.

Cartwright, A. (1979) *The Dignity of Labour: A Study of Childbearing and Induction.* London: Tavistock.

Cartwright, A. and O'Brien, M. (1976) Social class variation in health care and in the nature of general practitioner consultations. In Stacey, M. (ed.) *The Sociology of the NHS. Sociological Review Monograph* No. 22, University of Keele.

Cartwright, A. and Anderson, R. (1981) *General Practice Revisited: A Second Study of Patients and their Doctors.* London: Tavistock.

Cartwright, A., Shaw, S. and Spatley, T. (1975) *Designing a Comprehensive Community Response to Problems of Alcohol Abuse.* London: Maudsley Alcohol Pilot Project.

Central Statistical Office (1986) *Social Trends.* No. 16. London: HMSO.

Chamberlain, M. (1981) *Old Wives' Tales: their History, Remedies and Spells.* London: Virago.

Charlton, A. and Blair, V. (1989) Predicting the onset of smoking in boys and girls. *Social Science and Medicine*, **29**(7), 813–818.

Chavkin, W. (ed.) (1984) *Double Exposure – Women's Health Hazards on the Job and at Home.* New York: Monthly Review Press.

Chernin, K. (1983) *The Tyranny of Slenderness.* London: Women's Press.

Cherry, N. (1984a) Nervous strain, anxiety and symptoms among 32 year-old men at work in Britain. *Journal of Occupational Psychology*, **57**, 95–105.

Cherry, N. (1984b) Women and work-stress: evidence from the 1946 birth cohort. *Ergonomics*, **27**, 519–526.

Chesler, P. (1972) *Women and Madness.* New York: Doubleday.

Choiton, A., Spitzer, W. O., Roberts, S. R. *et al.* (1976) The patterns of medical drug use. *Canadian Medical Association Journal*, **114**, 33.

Clark, J. (1984) Mothers' perceptions of health visiting. *Health Visitor*, **57**, 265.

Clarke, J. N. (1983) Sexism, feminism and medicalism: a decade review of literature on gender and illness. *Sociology of Health and Ilness*, **5**(1), 62.

Clay, T. (1987) *Nurses, Power and Politics*. London: Heinemann.

Cleary, P. D. and Mechanic, D. (1983) Sex differences in psychological distress and married people. *Journal of Health and Social Behaviour*, **24**, 111–121.

Cohrane, R. and Stopes-Roe, M. (1981) Women, marriage, employment and mental health. *British Journal of Psychiatry*, **139**, 373-381.

Conrad, P. (1979) Types of medical social control. *Sociology of Health and Illness*, **1**(1), 1–11.

Conrad, P. (1981) On the medicalisation of deviance and social control. In Ingleby, D. (ed.) *Critical Psychiatry*. Harmondsworth: Penguin Books.

Cooper, C. L. and Marshall, T. (1976) Occupational sources of stress: a review of literature relating to coronary heart disease and mental ill health. *Journal of Occupational Psychology*, **49**, 11–28.

Cooperstock, R. (1978) Sex difference in psychotropic drug use. *Social Science and Medicine*, **12**(3B), 179–186.

Cooperstock, R. and Lennard, H. (1979) Some social meanings of tranquillizer use. *Sociology of Health and Illness*, **1**(3), 33.

Corbett, L. (1981) Getting our bodies back: menopausal self-help groups. *Women Wise*, **4**(1), 2–4.

Cornwell, J. (1984) *Hard Earned Lives – Accounts of Health and Illness from East London*. London and New York: Tavistock.

Corrigan, E. M. (1980) *Alcoholic Women in Treatment*. New York: Oxford University Press.

Corrigan, E. M. (1987) Women's combined use of alcohol and other mind-altering drugs. In Burden D. S. and Gottleib, N. (eds) *The Woman Client*. New York and London: Tavistock.

Cox, B. D. (ed.) (1987) *The Health and Life-style Survey*. London: Health-Promotion Research Trust.

Cradock, D. (1969) *Obesity and its Management*. London: Heinemann.

Crawford, M. and Hooper, D. (1973) Menopause, ageing in the family. *Social Science and Medicine*, **7**, 469–482.

Crull, P. (1982) The stress effects of sexual harassment on the job. *American Journal of Orthopsychiatry*, **52**(3), 539–544.

Crull, P. (1984) Sexual harassment and women's health. In Chavkin, W. (ed.) *Double Exposure – Women's Health Hazards on the Job and at Home*. New York: Monthly Review Press.

Currer, C. (1986) Concepts of mental well- and ill-being: the case of Pathan mothers in Britain. In Currer, C. and Stacey, M. (eds) *Concepts of Health, Illness and Disease – a Comparative Perspective*. Leamington Spa: Berg.

Cypress, B. K. (1984) *Patterns of Ambulatory Care in Obstetrics and Gynecology*. Hyattsville, M.D., US Department of Health and Human Services.

Davidson, M. J. and Cooper, C. L. (1981) A model of occupational stress. *Journal of Occupational Medicine*, **23**, 564–574.

Davies, C. (ed.) (1980) *Rewriting Nursing History*. London: Croom Helm.

Davis, F. (1963) *Passage Through Crisis*. Indianapolis: Bobbs-Merrill.

Dean, A. and Lin, N. (1977) The stress buffering role of social support. *Journal of Nervous and Mental Diseases*, **165**, 403-413.

De Jong, W. (1980) The stigma of obesity – the consequences of naive assumptions concerning the causes of physical deviance. *Health and Social Behaviour*, **21**(1), 75–87.

Department of Health and Social Security (1976) *Prevention and Health: Everybody's Business*. London: HMSO.

Department of Health and Social Security (1987) *Health and Personal Social Services Statistics for England*. London: HMSO.

Deutsch, H. (1944) *The Psychology of Women*. New York: Grune and Stratton.

Dight, S. E. (1976) *Scottish Drinking Habits*. Edinburgh: HMSO.

Dingwall, R., Eekelaar, J. M. and Murray, T. (1983) *The Protection of Children: State Intervention and Family Life*. Oxford: Blackwell.

Dobbs, J. and Marsh, A. (1984) *Smoking Among Secondary School Children*. London: OPCS.

Doll, W., Thompson, E. and Lefton, M. (1976) Beneath acceptance. *Social Science and Medicine*, **10**, 312–317.

Donnison, J. (1977) *Midwives and Medical Men: A History of Inter-Professional Rivalries and Women's Rights*. London: Heinemann.

Doyal, L. with Pennell, I. (1983) *The Political Economy of Health*. London: Pluto Press.

Doyal, L., Green, K., Irwin, A. *et al*. (1983) *Cancer in Britain: The Politics of Prevention*. London: Pluto Press.

Dunnell, K. and Cartwright, A. (1972) *Medicine Takers, Prescribers and Hoarders*. London: Routledge & Kegan Paul.

Durkheim, E. (1952) *Suicide*. London: Routledge & Kegan Paul.

Edgell, S. (1980) *Middle-class Couples*. London: Allen & Unwin.

Ehrenreich, B. and English, D. (1979) *For Her Own Good: 150 years of the Expert's Advice to Women*. London: Pluto Press.

Eisner, M. and Wright, M. (1986) A feminist approach to general practice. In Webb, C. (ed.) *Feminist Practice in Women's Health Care*. Chichester and New York: Wiley.

Engleman, E. G. (1974) Attitudes towards women physicians: a study of 500 clinic patients. *Western Journal of Medicine*, **120**, 95–100.

Evason, E. (1980) *Just Me and the Kids: A Study of Single Parent Families*. Belfast: Equal Opportunities Commission.

Evers, H. (1985) The frail elderly woman: emerging questions in ageing and women's health. In Lewin, E. and Oleson, V. (eds) *Women, Health and Healing*. London: Tavistock.

Everyman's Encyclopaedia (1967) Vol. **8**, p. 312. Medical Education. London: Dent.

Filmore, K. M. (1984) 'When angels fall': women's drinking as cultural preoccupation and as reality. In Wilsnack, S. C. and Beckman, L. J. (eds) *Alcohol Problems in Women*. New York: Guildford Press.

Finch, J. and Groves, D. (1983) *A Labour of Love: Women, Work and Caring*. London: Routledge & Kegan Paul.

Fink, P. J. (1980) Psychiatric myths of the menopause. In Eskin, L. (ed.) *The Menopause: Comprehensive Management*. New York: Nasson.

Fisher, S. and Groce, S. B. (1985) Doctor–patient negotiation of cultural assumptions. *Sociology of Health and Illness*, **7**(3), 342–374.

Flaherty, J. and Richman, J. (1989) Gender differences in the perception and utilization of social support: theoretical perspectives and an empirical test. *Social Science and Medicine*, **28**(12), 1221–1229.

Fleishman, J. (1984) The health hazards of office work. In Chavkin, W. (ed.) *Double Exposure – Women's Health Hazards on the Job and at Home*. New York: Monthly Review Press.

Fox, A. J. and Goldblatt, P. D. (1982) *OPCS Longitudinal Study: Socio-demographic Mortality Differentials 1971–75*. London: HMSO.

Freidson, E. (1975a) *Profession of Medicine – A Study of the Sociology of Applied Knowledge*. New York: Dodd, Mead.

Freidson, E. (1975b) Dilemmas in the doctor/patient relationship. In Cox, C. and Mead, A. (eds) *A Sociology of Medical Practice*. London: Collier Macmillan.

Freidson, E. (1986) *Professional Powers: A Study of the Institutionalisation of Formal Knowledge*. Chicago and London: University of Chicago Press.

Frey, K. (1981) Middle-aged women's experiences and perceptions of meno-pause. *Women and Health*, **6**(1–2), 25–36.

Funch, D. P. and Mettlin, C. (1982) The role of social support in relation to recovery from breast surgery. *Social Science and Medicine*, **16**, 91–8.

Game, A. and Pringle, R. (1984) *Gender at Work*. London: Pluto Press.

Ghodse, A. H. (1978) The attitudes of casualty staff and ambulance personnel towards patients who take drug overdoses. *Social Science and Medicine*, **12A**, 341.

Ginsberg, S. and Brown, G. B. (1982) No time for depression: a study of help-seeking among mothers of pre-school children. In Mechanic, D. (ed.) *Symptoms, Illness Behaviour and Help-seeking*. New York: Prodist.

Ginsberg, H. and Miller, S. (1982) Sex differences in children's risk-taking behaviour. *Child Development*, **53**, 426.

Goddard, E. and Ikin, C. (1986) *Smoking among Secondary Schoolchildren*. London: HMSO.

Goffman, E. (1963) *Stigma: Notes on the Management of Spoiled Identity*. Engle-wood Cliffs: Prentice-Hall.

Golding, J. (1987) Smoking. In Cox, B. D. (ed.) *The Health and Life-style Survey*. London: Health-Promotion Research Trust.

Gomberg, E. S. (1976) Alcoholism in women. In Kissin, B. and Beigleiter, H. (eds) *The Biology of Alcoholism*, Vol. 4. *Social Aspects of Alcoholism*. New York: Plenum.

Goodman, L. (1974) A report on children's toys. In Stacey, J., Daniels, J. and Bereaud, J. (eds) *And Jill Came Tumbling After*. New York: Dell.

Gordon, J. (1980) Women in medical school and beyond. *Medical Education*, **5**, 360–365.

Gove, W. R. (1972) The relationship between sex roles, mental illness and marital status. *Social Forces*, **51**, 34–44.

Gove, W. R. (1978) Sex differences in mental illness among men and women. *Social Science and Medicine*, **12** (3B), 187–198.

Gove, W. R. (1979) Sex differences in the epidemiology of mental dis-order: evidence and explanations. In Gomberg, E. S. and Franks, C. (eds) *Gender and Disordered Behaviour: Sex Differences in Psychopathology*. New York: Brunner/Hazel.

Gove, W. R. (1984) Gender differences in mental and physical illness: the effects of fixed roles and nurturant roles. *Social Science and Medicine,* **19**(2), 77–91.

Gove, W. R. and Tudor, F. (1973) Adult sex roles and mental illness. *American Journal of Sociology,* **78**, 812–835.

Gove, W. R. and Hughes, M. (1979) Possible causes of the apparent sex difference in physical health: an empirical investigation. *American Sociological Review,* **44**, 126–146.

Graham, H. (1983) Caring: a labour of love. In Finch, J. and Groves, C. (eds) *A Labour of Love.* London: Routledge & Kegan Paul.

Graham, H. (1984) *Women, Health and the Family.* Brighton: Wheatsheaf.

Graham, H. and Oakley, A. (1986) Competing ideologies of reproduction: medical and maternal perspectives on pregnancy. In Currer, C. and Stacey, M. (eds) *Concepts of Health, Illness and Disease.* Leamington Spa: Berg.

Grant, L. (1983) Peer expectations about outstanding competencies of men and women medical students. *Sociology of Health and Illness,* **5**(1), 42–61.

Gray, J. (1982) The effect of the doctor's sex on the doctor–patient relationship. *Journal of the Royal College of General Practitioners,* **32**, 167–169.

Grossman, H. Y., Salt, P., Nadelson, C. *et al.* (1987) Coping resources and health responses among men and women medical students. *Social Science and Medicine,* **25**(9), 1057–1063.

Gruber, J. and Bjorn, L. (1982) Blue collar blues: the sexual harassment of women autoworkers. *Work and Occupations,* **9**(3), 271–298.

Haar, E., Halitsky, V. and Stricker, G. (1975) Factors related to preferences for female gynaecologists. *Medical Care,* **13**, 782–790.

Haavio-Mannila, E. (1979) Development of sex differences in economic activity and mental health in Scandinavia. *Acta Sociologica,* **22**, 5–29.

Haavio-Mannila, E. (1986) Inequalities in health and gender. *Social Science and Medicine,* **22**(2), 141–149.

Haines, S. G. and Feinleib, M. (1980) Women, work and coronary heart disease. *American Journal of Public Health,* **70**, 133.

Harris, M. and Smith, S. (1983) The relationship of old age, sex, ethnicity and weight to stereotypes of obesity and self-perception. *International Journal of Obesity,* **7**, 361–371.

Harris, M., Harris, R. and Bochner, S. (1982) Fat, four-eyed and female – stereotypes of obesity, glasses and gender. *Journal of Applied Social Psychology,* **12**, 503–516.

Hart, N. (1976) *When Marriage Ends.* London: Tavistock.

Hart, N. (1988) Sex differentials and mortality in Europe. In Fox, A. J. (ed.) *Inequality in Health Within Europe.* Aldershot: Gower.

Heins, M. and Braslow, J. (1981) Women doctors: productivity in Great Britain and the United States. *Medical Education,* **15**, 53–56.

Heins, M., Hendricks, J. and Martindale, L. (1979) Attitudes of women and men physicians. *American Journal of Public Health,* **69**, 1132–1139.

Helman, C. (1981) Disease versus illness in general practice. *Journal of Royal College of General Practitioners,* **31**, 548.

Hemminki, E. (1974) General practitioners' indications for psychotropic drug therapy. *Scandinavian Journal of Social Medicine,* **2**, 1.

Hemminki, E., Pesonen, T. and Brown, K. (1981) Sales of psychotropic drugs in the Nordic countries. *Social Science and Medicine*, **15A**(5), 589–599.
Henderson, C. (1974) Care eliciting behaviour in man. *Journal of Nervous Mental Diseases*, **159**, 172–181.
Henderson, C., Byrne, D. G., Duncan-Jones, P. *et al.* (1980) Social relationships, adversity and neurosis. *British Journal of Psychiatry*, **136**, 574–584.
Henifin, M. S. (1984) The particular problems of video display terminals. In Chavkin, W. (ed.) *Double Exposure*. New York: Monthly Review Press.
Herzlich, C. (1973) *Health and Illness*. London and New York: Academic Press.
Herzlich, C. and Pierret, J. (1986) Illness: from causes to meaning. In Currer, C. and Stacey, M. (eds) *Concepts of Health, Illness and Disease – A Comparative Perspective*. Leamington Spa: Berg.
Hibbard, J. H. and Pope, C. R. (1983) Gender roles, illness orientation and use of medical services. *Social Science and Medicine*, **17**(3), 129–137.
Hirsch, B. J. (1979) Psychological dimensions of social network: a multimethod analysis. *American Journal of Sociology*, 812–835.
Hoferek, M. J. and Sarnowski, A. (1981) Feelings of loneliness in women medical students. *Journal of Medical Education*, **56**, 397.
Homans, H. (1985) Discomforts in pregnancy: traditional remedies and medical prescriptions. In Homans, H. (ed.) *The Sexual Politics of Reproduction*. Aldershot and Brookfield: Gower.
Homans, H. (1987) Man-made myths: the reality of being a woman scientist in the NHS. In Spencer, A. and Podmore, D. (eds) *In a Man's World*. London and New York: Tavistock.
Homans, H. and Satow, A. (1981) We too are strangers. *Journal of Community Nursing*, November.
Homans, H. and Satow, A. (1982) Can you hear me? Cultural variations in communication. *Journal of Community Nursing*, January.
Hopkins, I. K. G. (1980) Psychiatric illness following childbirth: are husbands an etiological factor? *Social Science and Medicine*, **14A**, 621–626.
Hopper, S. (1981) Diabetes as a stigmatising condition. *Social Science and Medicine*, **15B**, 11–19.
Horwitz, A. (1977) The pathways into psychiatric treatment: some differences between men and women. *Journal of Health and Social Behaviour*, **18**, 169–178.
House, J. S., Robbins, C. and Metzner, H. L. (1982) The association of social relationships and activities to mortality: prospective evidence from Tecumseh Community Health Study. *American Journal of Epidemiology*, **116**, 123–140.
Hughes, D. (1988) When nurse knows best: some aspects of nurse/doctor interaction in a casualty department. *Sociology of Health and Illness*, **10**, 1.
Hunt, S., McEwan, J. and McKenna, S. (1985) Social inequalities and perceived health effect. *Health Care*, **2**, 151.
Huppert, F. (1987) in Cox, B. D. (ed.) *The Health and Life-style Survey*, London: Health-Promotion Research Trust.
Hutt, R., Parsons, D. and Pearson, R. (1981) The timing of and reasons for doctors' career decisions. *Health Trends*, **13**, 17–20.
Illich, I. (1977) *Limits to Medicine*. Harmondsworth: Penguin Books.
Jefferys, M. and Sachs, H. (1983) *Rethinking General Practice*. London and New York: Tavistock.

Jerome, D. (1981) The significance of friendship for women in later life. *Ageing and Society*, **1**, 175–197.

Jobling, R. (1988) The experience of psoriasis under treatment. In Anderson, R. and Bury, M. (eds) *Living with Chronic Illness*. London and Boston: Unwin Hyman.

Kadushin, C. (1968) *Why People Go to Psychiatrists?* New York: Atherton.

Karpf, A. (1988) *Doctoring the Media: The Reporting of Health and Medicine*. London and New York: Routledge.

Kaufert, P. (1981) Symptom reporting at menopause. *Social Science and Medicine*, **15E**(3), 173–185.

Kaufert, P. (1982) Myth and the menopause. *Sociology of Health and Illness*, **4**, 141–166.

Kaufert, P. (1984) Women and their health in the middle years: A Manitoba Project. *Social Science and Medicine*, **18** (3), 279–281.

Kaufert, P. and McKinley, S. M. (1985) Estrogen-replacement therapy. In Lewin, E. and Olesen, V. (eds) *Women, Health and Healing*. New York and London: Tavistock.

Kaufert, P. and Gilbert, P. (1986a) Women, menopause and medicalisation. *Culture, Medicine and Psychiatry*, **10**, 7–21.

Kaufert, P. and Gilbert, P. (1986b) The context of menopause: psychotropic drug use and menopausal status. *Social Science; and Medicine*, **23**(8), 747–755.

Kelly, J. M. (1980) Sex preference in patient selection of a family physician. *Journal of Family Practitioners*, **11**, 427.

Kessler, R. (1985) Social factors in psychopathology: stress, social support and coping processes. *American Review of Psychology*, **36**, 531–572.

Klerman, G. L. (1978) Stress, Adaptation and Affective Disorders. Paper presented to the American Psychopathological Association, Boston, March, 1978.

King, J. (1987) Well Woman Centres. Unpublished Report, University of Southampton.

Kirke, P. N. (1980) Mothers' views of obstetric care. *British Journal of Obstetrics and Gynaecology*, **87**, 1029–1033.

Knupfer, G. (1982) *Problems Associated with Drunkenness in Women*. Alcohol and Health Monograph 4. Rockville, MD: NIAAA.

Komarovsky, M. (1967) *Blue Collar Marriage*. New York: Vintage Books.

Koos, E. L. (1954) *The Health of Regionville*. New York: Columbia University Press.

Korman, M. and Stubblefield, R. (1971) Medical school evaluation of internship performance. *Journal of Medical Education*, **46**, 670–673.

Koumjian, K. (1981) The use of Valium as a form of social control. *Social Science and Medicine*, **15E**, 245.

Kumar, R. and Robson, K. M. (1984) A prospective study of emotional disorders in childbearing women. *British Journal of Psychiatry*, **144**, 35–47.

Laing, R. D. (1967) *The Politics of Experience*. Harmondsworth: Penguin.

Land, H. (1981) *Parity Begins at Home*. Manchester: EDC.

Langwell, K. M. (1982) Differences by sex in economic returns with physician specialization. *Journal of Health Politics, Policy and Law*, **6**, 752–761.

Larkin, G. (1981) Professional autonomy and the ophthalmic optician. *Sociology of Health and Illness*, **3**(1), 15–30.

Larkin, G. (1983) *Occupational Monopoly and Modern Medicine*. London and New York: Tavistock.

Lawrence, B. (1987) The fifth dimension – gender and general practice. In Spencer, A. and Podmore, D. (eds) *In a Man's World*. London and New York: Tavistock.

Laws, S. (1985) Male power and menstrual etiquette. In Homans, H. (ed.) *The Sexual Politics of Reproduction*. Aldershot: Gower.

Leeson, J. and Gray, J. (1978) *Women and Medicine*. London: Tavistock.

Leichner, P. and Harper, D. (1982) Sex role ideology among physicians. *Canadian Medical Association Journal*, **127**, 380.

Leighton, A. H. (1984) Barriers to adequate care for mentally ill people. *Social Science and Medicine*, **18**(3), 237.

Lennane, J. K. and Lennane, R. J. (1973) Alleged psychogenic disorders in women – a possible manifestation of sexual prejudice. *New England Journal of Medicine*, **288**, 6.

Leserman, J. (1981) *Men and Women in Medical School*. New York: Praeger.

Leviathan, U. and Cohen, J. (1985) Gender differences in life expectancy among kibbutz members. *Social Science and Medicine*, **21**(5), 545–551.

Lobban, G. (1978) The influence of the school on sex-role stereotyping. In Chetwynd, J. and Harnett, O. (eds) *The Sex Role System*. London: Routledge and Kegan Paul.

Lopez, A. D. (1984) Sex differentials in mortality. *WHO Chronicle*, **38**(5), 317–324.

Lorber, J. (1975) Good patients and problem patients: conformity and deviance in a general hospital. *Journal of Health and Social Behaviour*, **16**, 213–225.

Lorber, J. (1984) *Women Physicians – Careers, Status and Power*. London: Tavistock.

Macfarlane, A. and Mugford, M. (1984) *Birth Counts: Statistics of Pregnancy and Childbirth*. Vols. 1 and 2. London: HMSO.

Macintyre, S. (1977a) *Single and Pregnant*. London: Croom Helm.

Macintyre, S. (1977b) Old age as a social problem: historical notes on the English experience. In Dingwall, R. (ed.) *Health Care and Health Knowledge*. London: Croom Helm.

Macintyre, S. (1986) The patterning of health by social position in contemporary Britain: directions for sociological research. *Social Science and Medicine*, **23**(4), 393.

Macintyre, S. and Oldman, D. (1977) Coping with migraine. In Davis, A. and Horobin, G. (eds) *Medical Encounters*. London: Croom Helm.

Maclean, U. (1974) *Nursing in Contemporary Society*. London: Routledge & Kegan Paul.

MacPherson, K. (1981) Menopause as disease – the social construction of a metaphor. *Advances in Nursing Science*, **3**(2), 95.

Marcus, A. C. and Seeman, T. E. (1981) Sex differences in health status: a re-examination of the nurturant role hypothesis. *American Sociological Review*, **46**, 119.

Marcus, A. C., Seeman, T. E. and Telesky, C. W. (1983) Sex differences in reports of illness and disability: a further test of the fixed role hypothesis. *Social Science and Medicine*, **17**(15), 993.

Mares, P., Henley, A. and Baxter, C. (1985) *Health Care in Multiracial Britain.* Cambridge: Health Education Council.

Margolis, A. J., Greenwood, S. and Heilbron, D. (1983) Survey of men and women residents entering United States obstetrics and gynaecology programs in 1981. *American Journal of Obstetrics and Gynecology*, **146**, 541.

Marieskind, H. (1980) *Women in the Health System: Patients, Providers and Programs,* St Louis: C. V. Mosby.

Marsden, D. (1973) *Mothers Alone: Poverty and the Fatherless Family.* Harmondsworth: Penguin.

Martin, E. (1989) *The Woman in the Body – A Cultural Analysis of Reproduction.* Milton Keynes: Open University Press.

Martin, J. and Roberts, C. (1984) *Women and Employment: A Lifetime Perspective.* London: HMSO.

Martin, R. and Wallace, J. (1985) Women and unemployment: activities and social contact. In Roberts, B., Finnegan, R. and Gallie, D. (eds) *New Approaches to Economic Life.* Manchester: University Press.

Martin, S. (1989) PhD thesis, University of Southampton.

McCranie, E. W., Horowitz, A. J. and Martin, R. (1978) Alleged sex-role stereotyping in the assessment of women's physical complaints: A study of general practitioners. *Social Science and Medicine*, **12**, 111.

McKinley, S. and McKinley, J. (1985) Health status and health care utilisation by menopausal women. In McKinley, S. and McKinley, J. (eds) *Ageing, Reproduction and the Climacteric.* New York: Plenum.

Mead, M. (1935) *Sexual Temperament in Three Primitive Societies,* New York: W. Morow.

Mechanic, D. (1968) *Medical Sociology.* New York: The Free Press. London: Macmillan.

Mechanic, D. (1982) The epidemiology of illness behaviour and its relationship to physical and psychological distress. In Mechanic, D. (ed.) *Symptoms, Illness Behaviour and Help-seeking.* New York: Prodist.

Meininger, J. (1986) Sex differences in factors associated with use of medical care and alternative illness behaviour. *Social Science and Medicine*, **22**(3), 285.

Merrison, A. (1979) *A Report of the Royal Commission on the National Health Service.* London: HMSO.

Merton, R. K., Reader, G. and Kendall, P. (1957) *The Student Physician.* Cambridge, Mass.: Harvard University Press.

Miles, A. (1978) The social content of health. In Brearley, P., Gibbons, J., Miles, A. *et al.* (eds) *The Social Context of Health Care.* London: Martin Robertson.

Miles, A. (1979) Some psychosocial consequences of multiple sclerosis: a study of group identity. *British Journal of Medical Psychology*, **52**, 321.

Miles, A. (1984) The stigma of psychiatric disorder: a sociological perspective and research report. In Reed, J. and Lomas, G. (eds) *Psychiatric Services in the Community.* London: Croom Helm.

Miles, A. (1987) *The Mentally Ill in Contemporary Society.* Oxford: Blackwell.

Miles, A. (1988) *Women and Mental Illness.* Brighton: Wheatsheaf.

Miller, S. (1983) *Men and Friendship.* Boston, Mass: Houghton Mifflin.

Miller, P. and Ingham, J. G. (1976) Friends, confidants and symptoms. *Social Psychiatry*, **11**, 51.

Milliren, J. W. (1977) Some contingencies affecting the utilization of tranquillizers in long-term care of the elderly. *Journal of Health and Social Behaviour*, **18**, 206.

Millum, T. (1975) *Images of Women: Advertising in Women's Magazines*. London: Chatto & Windus.

Mitchell, J. and Oakley, A. (1986) *What is Feminism?* Oxford: Blackwell.

Morgan, D. (1985) *The Family, Politics and Social Theory*. London: Routledge.

Morgan, J. (1988) Living with renal failure on home haemodialysis. In Anderson, R. and Bury, M. (eds) *Living with Chronic Illness*. London and Boston: Unwin Hyman.

Morgan, M. (1980) Marital status, health, illness and service use. *Social Science and Medicine*, **14A**, 633.

Morsy, S. A. (1978) Sex differences and folk illness in an Egyptian village. In Beck, I. and Keddie, R. (eds) *Women in the Muslim World*. Cambridge. Mass.: Harvard University Press.

Moss, E. and Davidson, S. (1982) Attitudes towards mental illness in a sample of Israeli rehabilitation workers. *International Journal of Rehabilitation Research*, **5**, 45.

Mueller, D. (1980) Social networks: a promising direction for research on the relationship of the social environment to psychiatric disorder. *Social Science and Medicine*, **14A**(2), 147.

Mumford, E. (1983) *Medical Sociology*. New York: Random House.

Murcott, A. (1982) It's a pleasure to cook for him: food, mealtimes and gender in some South Wales households. In Garmanikov, E., Morgan, D., Purvis, J. *et al.* (eds) *The Public and the Private*. London: Heinemann.

Murcott, A. (1983) Cooking and the cooked. In Murcott, A. (ed.) *The Sociology of Food and Eating*. Aldershot: Gower.

Nathanson, C. A. (1975) Illness and the feminine role: a theoretical review. *Social Science and Medicine*, **2**, 57.

Nathanson, C. A. (1977) Sex, Illness and Medical Care: A Review of Data, Theory and Method. *Social Science and Medicine*, **11**, 13.

Nathanson, C. A. (1980) Social roles and health status among women: the significance of employment. *Social Science and Medicine*, **14A**(6), 463.

National Council of Women (1976) *Report of a Working Party on Alcohol Problems in Women and Young People*. London: National Council of Women.

Navarro, V. (1976) *Medicine Under Capitalism*. New York: Prodist.

Newton, P. (1987) Who becomes an engineer? – social-psychological antecedents of a non-traditional career choice. In Spencer, A. and Podmore, D. (eds) *In a Man's World*. London: Tavistock.

Nicolson, P. (1986) Developing a feminist approach to depression following childbirth. In Wilkinson, S. (ed.) *Feminist Social Psychology: Developing Theory and Practice*. Milton Keynes: Open University Press.

Oakley, A. (1974) *Housewife*. London: Allen Lane.

Oakley, A. (1981) *From Here to Maternity – Becoming a Mother*. Harmondsworth: Penguin.

Oakley, A. (1982) *Subject Women*. Glasgow: Fontana Paperbacks.

Oakley, A. (1984a) *The Captured Womb: A History of the Medical Care of Pregnant Women.* Oxford: Blackwell.

Oakley, A. (1984b) The importance of being a nurse. *Nursing Times,* January 10.

Oakley, A. (1986) Feminism, motherhood and medicine – who cares? In Mitchell, J. and Oakley, A. (eds) *What is Feminism?* Oxford: Blackwell.

Oakley, A., McPherson, A. and Roberts, H. (1984) *Miscarriage.* Glasgow: Fontana Paperbacks.

O'Brien, G. E. (1984) Reciprocal effects between locus of control and job attributes. *Australian Journal of Psychology,* **35**, 461.

Office of Health Economics: (1987) *Women's Health Today.* London: OHE.

Office of Population Censuses and Surveys (1986) *General Household Survey for 1985.* OPCS Monitor.

Open University (1985) *Studying Health and Disease.* Milton Keynes: Open University Press.

Orbach, S. (1978) *Fat Is a Feminist Issue.* London: Paddington Press.

Orbach, S. (1986) *Hungerstrike.* London and Boston: Faber & Faber.

Organization for Economic Co-operation and Development (1985) *The Integration of Women into the Economy.* Paris: OECD.

Orr, J. (1986) Feminism and health visiting. In Webb, C. (ed.) *Feminist Practice in Women's Health Care.* Chichester and New York: Wiley.

Ovretveit, J. (1985) Medical dominance and the development of professional autonomy in physiotherapy. *Sociology of Health and Illness,* **7**(1), 76.

Parsons, T. (1951) Social Structure and dynamic process: the case of modern medical practice. In Parsons, T. (ed.) *The Social System.* New York: Free Press.

Parsons, T. (1958) Definitions of health and illness in the light of American values and social structure. In Jaco, E. G. (ed.) *Patients, Physicians and Illness.* New York: Free Press.

Passannante, M. R. and Nathanson, C. A. (1985) Female labor force participation and female mortality in Wisconsin 1974–1978. *Social Science and Medicine,* **21**(6), 655.

Paykel, E. S., Emms, E. M., Fletcher, T. *et al.* (1980) Life events and social support in puerperal depression. *British Journal of Psychiatry,* **136**, 339.

Phillips, A. and Rakusen, J. (1978) *Our Bodies, Ourselves – a Health Book by and for Women.* Harmondsworth: Penguin.

Pilisuk, M. and Froland, C. (1978) Kinship, social networks, social support and health. *Social Science and Medicine,* **12B**, 237.

Pill, R. and Stott, N. (1982) Concepts of illness causation and responsibility: some preliminary data from a sample of working class mothers. *Social Science and Medicine,* **16**, 43–52.

Pinder, R. (1988) Striking balance: living with Parkinson's disease. In Anderson, R. and Bury, M. (eds) *Living with Chronic Illness.* London and Boston: Unwin Hyman.

Popay, J., Rimmer, L. and Rossiter, C. (1983) *One Parent Families: Parents, Children and Public Policy.* London: Study Commission on the Family.

Porter, M. and Macintyre, S. (1984) What is, must be best: A research note on conservative or deferential responses to antenatal care provision. *Social Science and Medicine,* **19**(11), 1197-1200.

Preston-Whyte, M. E., Fraser, R. C. and Beckett, J. L. (1983) Effect of a principal's gender on consultation patterns. *Journal of the Royal College of General Practitioners,* **33**, 654–658.

Rahav, M., Struening, E. L. and Andrew, H. (1984) Opinions on mental illness in Israel. *Social Science and Medicine,* **19**, 115.

Richards, J., Calkins, E., McCanse, A. *et al.* (1974) Predicting performance in a combined undergraduate and medical education program. *Educational and Psychological Measurement,* **34**, 923–931.

Richman, A. and Bury, A. (1985) More and more is less and less: the myth of massive psychiatric need. *British Journal of Psychiatry,* **146**, 164.

Riesman, C. K. (1983) Women and medicalisation: a new perspective. *Social Policy,* 3–18.

Roberts, H. (1985) *The Patient Patients: Women and their Doctors.* London: Pandora.

Robinson, D. (1971) *The Process of Becoming Ill.* London: Routledge & Kegan Paul.

Robinson, D. (1979) *Alcohol Problems.* London: Macmillan.

Robinson, I. (1988) Reconstructing lives: negotiating the meaning of multiple sclerosis. In Anderson, R. and Bury, M. (eds) *Living with Chronic Illness.* London and Boston: Unwin Hyman.

Romalis, S. (1985) Struggle between providers and recipients: the case of birth practices. In Lewin, E. and Olesen, V. (eds) *Women, Health and Healing.* New York and London: Tavistock.

Rosenberg, M. G. (1984) The home is the workplace. In Chavkin, W. (ed.) *Double Exposure.* New York: Monthly Review Press.

Rosenblatt, A. and Kirk, S. (1982) Social roles of women in medicine, psychiatry and social work. *American Journal of Orthopsychiatry,* **52**, 430–439.

Royal College of General Practitioners (1986) *Morbidity Statistics from General Practice 1981–82. Third National Survey.* London: HMSO.

Royal Commission on Medical Education (Todd Report) (1968) *Cmnd 3569.* London: HMSO.

Ruzek, S. B. (1978) *Women's Health Movement: Feminist Alternatives to Medical Control.* New York: Praeger.

Salvage, J. (1985) *The Politics of Nursing.* London: Heinemann.

Sargent, M. (1979) *Drinking and Alcoholism in Australia: A Power Relation Theory.* Melbourne: Longmans.

Saunders, B. (1980) Psychological aspects of women and alcohol. In *Camberwell Council on Alcoholism: Women and Alcohol.* London: Tavistock.

Scadron, A., Witte, M. H., Axelrod, M. and Greenberg, E. (1982) Attitudes toward women physicians in medical academia. *Journal of the American Medical Association,* **247**(20), 2803.

Scambler, A. and Scambler, G. (1985) Menstrual symptoms, attitudes and consulting behaviour. *Social Science and Medicine,* **20**(10), 1065–1068.

Scambler, G. and Hopkins, A. (1988) Accommodating epilepsy in families. In Anderson, R. and Bury, M. (eds) *Living with Chronic Illness.* London and Boston: Unwin Hyman.

Scheff, T. (1966) *Being Mentally Ill – A Sociological Theory.* Chicago: Aldine.

Scully, D. (1980) *Men Who Control Women's Health: The Miseducation of Obstetricians and Gynecologists.* Boston: Houghton Mifflin.

Seabrook, J. (1986) The unprivileged: a hundred years of their ideas about health and illness. In Currer, C. and Stacey, M. (eds) *Concepts of Health, Illness and Disease – A Comparative Perspective.* Leamington Spa: Berg.

Shapiro, M. C., Najman, J. M., Chang, A. *et al.* (1983) Information control and the exercise of power in the obstetric encounter. *Social Science and Medicine,* **17**(3), 139–146.

Sharpe, S. (1984) *Double Identity.* Harmondsworth: Penguin.

Shaw, S. (1980) The causes of increasing drinking problems amongst women: a general aetiological theory. In *Camberwell Council on Alcoholism: Women and Alcohol.* London: Tavistock.

Shearer, A. (1981) *Disability: Whose Handicap?* Oxford: Blackwell.

Shimmin, S., McNally, J. and Liff, S. (1981) Pressures on women engaged in factory work. *Employment Gazette,* August, 344–349.

Shorter, E. (1984) *A History of Women's Bodies.* Harmondsworth: Penguin.

Shuttle, P. and Redgrove, P. (1986) *The Wise Wound.* London: Paladin.

Skultans, V. (1970) The symbolic significance of menstruation and the menopause. *Man,* **5**(4), 639–651.

Smith, A. (1968) *The Science of Social Medicine.* London: Staples.

Smith, D. and David, S. J. (eds) (1975) *Women Look at Psychiatry.* Vancouver: Press Gang.

Snowden, R. and Christian, B. (eds) (1983) *Patterns and Perceptions of Menstruation – a WHO International Study.* Beckenham: Croom Helm.

Spencer, A. and Podmore, D. (1987) Women lawyers – marginal members of a male-dominated profession. In Spencer, A. and Podmore, D. (eds) *In a Man's World: Essays on Women in Male-dominated Professions.* London: Tavistock.

Spencer, N. J. (1984) Parents' recognition of the ill child. In Macfarlane, J. A. (ed.) *Progress in Child Health.* Edinburgh: Churchill-Livingstone.

Spiegel, D. A., Smolen, R. C. and Jonas, C. K. (1986) An examination of the relationship among interpersonal stress, morale and academic performance in male and female medical students. *Social Science and Medicine,* **23**(11), 1157–1161.

Stacey, M. (1988) *The Sociology of Health and Healing.* London: Unwin Hyman.

Stark, J. (1987) Health and social contacts. In Cox, B. D. (ed.) *The Health and Life-style Survey.* London: Health-Promotion Research Trust.

Stellman, J. H. (1977) *Women's Work, Women's Health: Myths and Realities.* New York: Pantheon.

Stellman, J. H. (1978) Occupational health hazards of women: an overview. *Preventive Medicine,* **7**, 281–293.

Stephen, P. J. (1987) Career patterns of women medical graduates 1974–84. *Medical Education,* **21**, 255–259.

Stimson, G. (1976) General practitioners, 'trouble' and types of patient. In: Stacey, M. (ed.) *The Sociology of the NHS. Sociological Review Monographs* no. 22. Keele: University of Keele.

Stimson, G. and Webb, B. (1975) *Going To See the Doctor: The Consultation Process in General Practice.* London and Boston: Routledge & Kegan Paul.

Stone, A. A. and Neal, J. M. (1984) New measures of daily coping: development and preliminary results. *Journal of Personal Social Psychology,* **46**, 892–896.

Stroebe, M. S. and Stroebe, W. (1983) Who suffers more? Sex differences in health risks of the widowed. *Psychological Bulletin*, **93**, 279–301.

Strong, P. M. (1979) Sociological imperialism and the profession of medicine. *Social Science and Medicine*, **13A**(2), 199–215.

Sudnow, D. (1967) *Passing On – The Social Organisation of Dying*. New Jersey: Prentice-Hall.

Sullivan, D. A. and Beeman, R. (1982) Satisfaction with maternity care: a matter of communication and choice. *Medical Care*, **20**(3), 321.

Szasz, T. (1961) *The Myth of Mental Illness*. New York: Harper.

Szasz, T. (1971) *The Manufacture of Madness*. London: Routledge.

Taylor, W. C. (1871) *A Physician's Counsels to Women in Health and Disease*. Springfield: Holland & Co.

Teperi, J. and Rimpela, M. (1989) Menstrual pain, health and behaviour in girls. *Social Science and Medicine*, **29**(2), 163–169.

Thoits, P. A. (1983) Dimensions of life-events that influence psychological distress. In Kaplan, H.B. (ed.) *Psychosocial Stress: Trends in Theory and Research*. New York: Academic Press.

Townsend, P. and Davidson, N. (1982) *Inequalities in Health*, London: Penguin.

Tuckett, D. (1976) *An Introduction to Medical Sociology*. London: Tavistock.

Tuckett, D., Boulton, M., Olson, C. *et al.* (1985) *Meetings Between Experts*. London and New York: Tavistock.

Turner, B. (1987) *Medical Power and Social Knowledge*. London: Sage.

Ungerson, C. (1987) *Policy Is Personal: Sex, Gender and Informal Care*. London and New York: Tavistock.

United Nations (1981) *Demographic Yearbook*. New York: United Nations.

United States Department of Health, Education and Welfare (1979) *Smoking and Health – A Report of the Surgeon General*. Washington DC.: DHEW No. 79–500 66.

United States Department of Labor (1977) *Working Women: A Data Book*. Washington: Government Printing Office.

Vaughn, C. E. and Leff, J. P. (1976) The influence of family and social factors on the course of psychiatric illness. *British Journal of Psychiatry*, **129**, 125–137.

Veevers, J. (1982) Women in driver's seat: trends in sex differences in driving and death. *Population Research Policy Review (Washington)*, **1**, 171.

Venters, M. (1981) Familial coping with chronic and severe childhood illness: the case of cystic fibrosis. *Social Science and Medicine*, **15A**, 289–297.

Verbrugge, L. M. (1976) Sex differentials in morbidity and mortality in the United States. *Social Biology*, **23**, 275.

Verbrugge, L. M. (1981) Recent trends in sex mortality differentials in the United States. *Women and Health*, **5**, 17–37.

Verbrugge, L. M. (1982) Sex differentials in health. *Public Health Reports*, **97**, 417.

Verbrugge, L. M. (1983) Multiple roles and physical health of women and men. *Journal of Health and Social Behaviour*, **24**, 16.

Verbrugge, L. M. (1986) From sneezes to adieux: stages of health for American men and women. *Social Science and Medicine*, **22**(11), 1195–1212.

Verbrugge, L. M. and Steiner, R. P. (1981) Physician treatment of men and women patients: sex bias or appropriate care? *Medical Care*, **19**(6), 609.

Vernoff, J., Douvan, E. and Kulka, R. (1981) *The Inner American*. New York: Basic Books.

Versluysen, M. C. (1980) Old wives' tales? Women healers in English history. In Davis, C. (ed.) *Rewriting Nursing History*. London: Croom Helm.

Waldron, I. (1976) Why do women live longer than men? *Social Science and Medicine*, **10**, 349.

Waldron, I. (1980) Employment and women's health: an analysis of causal relationships. *International Journal of Health Service*, **10**, 435–454.

Waldron, I. (1982a) An analysis of causes of sex differences in mortality and morbidity. In Gove, W. and Carpenter, G. (eds.) *The Fundamental Connection Between Nature and Nurture*. Lexington: Lexington Books.

Waldron, I. (1982b) Gender, psychophysiological disorders and mortality. In Al-Issa, I. (ed.) *Gender and Psychopathology*. New York: Academic Press.

Waldron, I. (1983a) Sex differences in human mortality: the role of genetic factors. *Social Science and Medicine*, **17**, 321–333.

Waldron, I. (1983b) Sex differences in illness incidence, prognosis and mortality. *Social Science and Medicine*, **17**(16), 1107-1123.

Walker, G. (1975) Social network in rural space. *East Lakes Geographer*, **10**, 68–77.

Walkerdine, V. (1984) Some day my prince will come. In McRobbie, A. and Nava, M. (eds) *Gender and Generation*. London: Macmillan.

Wallen, J., Waitzkin, H. and Stoeckle, J. D. (1979) Physician stereotypes about female health and illness. *Women and Health*, **4**, 135–146.

Walters, P. (1987) Servants of the Crown. In Spencer, A. and Podmore, D. (eds) *In A Man's World: Essays on Women in Male-dominated Professions*. London: Tavistock.

Wansbrough, N. and Cooper, P. (1980) *Open Employment After Mental Illness*. London: Tavistock.

Ward, A. W. M. (1982) Careers of medical women. *British Medical Journal*, **284**, 31.

Warr, P. (1987) *Work, Unemployment and Mental Health*. Oxford: Clarendon Press.

Warr, P. and Parry, G. (1982) Paid employment and women's psychological well-being. *Psychological Bulletin*, **91**, 498-516.

Webb, C. (1986) Women as gynaecology patients and nurses. In Webb, C. (ed.) *Feminist Practices in Women's Health Care*. Chichester and New York: Wiley.

Webb, C. and Wilson-Barnett, J. (1983) Coping with hysterectomy. *Journal of Advanced Nursing*, **8**(3), 311–319.

Weisman, C. S. and Tetelbaum, M. A. (1985) Physician gender and the physician patient relationship: recent evidence and relevant questions. *Social Science and Medicine*. **20**, 11.

Weissman, M. and Klerman, G. L. (1977) Sex differences and the epidemiology of depression. *Archives of General Psychiatry*, **24**, 98–111.

Welch, S. and Booth, A. (1977) Employment and health among married women with children. *Sex Roles*, **33**, 385–397.

Wenger, G. C. (1984) *The Supportive Network: Coping With Old Age*. London: Allen & Unwin.

Whitehead, M. (1988) *The Health Divide: Inequalities in Health in the 1980s*. Harmondsworth: Penguin.

Whittington, H. J. (1977) Widowhood in a Seaside Resort. M.Litt. thesis, University of Lancaster.

Wiles, R. (1990) Draft PhD thesis, to be submitted to the University of Southampton.

Wood, G. (1983) *The Myth of Neurosis*. London: Macmillan.

Wooley, S. and Wooley, O. (1979) Obesity and Women. I. – A closer look at the facts. *Women's Studies International Quarterly*, **2**, 69–79.

Wooley, O., Wooley, S. and Dyrenforth, S. (1979) Obesity and women. II. – a neglected feminist topic. *Women's Studies International Quarterly*, **2**, 81–92.

World Health Organization Scientific Group (1981) Research on the Menopause. Geneva: WHO.

Yarrow, M., Clausen, J. A. and Robbins, P. (1955) The social meaning of mental illness. *Journal of Social Issues*, **11**, 33–48.

Young, G. (1981) A woman in medicine – reflections from the inside. In Roberts, H. (ed.) *Women, Health and Reproduction*. London: Routledge & Kegan Paul.

Zola, I. K. (1971) Paper presented at the Medical Sociology Conference of the British Medical Association, November 1971, at Weston-super-Mare.

Zola, I. K. (1975) Medicine as an institution of social control. In Cox, C. and Mead, A. (eds) *A Sociology of Medical Practice*. London: Collier Macmillan.

Author index

Subject index

health professions, *see also* doctors, GPs,
    health visitors, hospital medical staff,
    midwives and nurses
health visitors, attitude, 170–2
    and sex stereotyping, 141–2
heart disease,
    and smoking, 27
    and women, 10
homosexuality as an illness, 184
hormone replacement therapy, 198
Hospital In-Patient Enquiry, 2
hospital medical staff
    and gender, 143
    and grades, 143–4
housewife as a role, 90
housewives,
    and alcohol consumption, 35–6
    and ill health, 16
    and mortality, 16
housing, 183
    and health, 13–14
    and single mothers, 26
Hungary, doctors, 132
husbands as carers, 101–3
    as emotional support, 96–7
hyperactivity, 202–3
hypertension, consultation rates, 8
hysterectomy, 97, 98, 178

ill-health, patterns of 1–12
    and working mothers, 17–19
illness,
    advice sources, 70–1
    concept of, 3–4, 42–3
    and gender differences, 44–5
    and occupational stress, 20, 21–2
    perceived causes 43–53
    and single mothers, 25–6
illness behaviour,
    and ethnic origin, 59, 62
    and gender, 58–62
    and social class, 59, 62, 68–9
illness, chronic and stigma, 110–23, 197
illness profile, 9
illness scores, 8
    and single mothers, 26
India,
    attitude to menstruation, 55–6, 78
    life expectancy, 6
    medical consultation, 63
Indonesia, attitude to menstruation, 55
infection as cause of illness, 44
infectious diseases and women, 10
internal medicine and women doctors, 144
International Classification of Diseases (ICD),
    2
Israel, Kibbutz society effect of, 11–12

Jamaica, attitude to menstruation, 55
Japan and medical consultation, 63
    and women in labour force, 15

Korea, women and menstruation, 78

labour division of in health professions,
    124–58
life expectancy, 5

malignant neoplasms, *see* cancer
marital problems, 204–5
marital status,
    and alcohol consumption, 35
    and health, 13
    and ill health, 24–5
    and psychiatric illness, 186–7
    and smoking, 30
    and stress, 25–6
medical consultation, *see* consultation
medical education, 133–49
medical information, access to, 177–81
medical schools,
    American, 135–6
    Australian, 135–6
    Canadian, 136
    and gender, 134
medical students,
    and alcohol abuse, 139
    expectations of, 137–40
    and social class, 59, 62, 68–9
    type casting, 137–40
medical specialties and gender, 144–7
medical treatment, side effects, 178
medicine and social control, 182–5
menopause, 117–120
    as a health problem, 42, 53
    and lay advice, 70
    medicalization of, 197–8
menstruation, 117
    in Finnish women, 84
    as a health problem, 42
    as illness, 53–7
    and Indian & Korean women, 78
    and Indonesian, Jamaican, Pakistani and
        Phillipino women, 55
    and medical consultation, 66
    and taboo, 56
    WHO survey, 54–6
mental handicap and women doctors, 144,
    147
mental illness,
    concept of in US, 43
    and education, 43
    and social class, 43
    as stigma, 43, 108–9
mental illness *see also* anxiety, depression and
    psychiatric illness